Assessing Dangerousness

JACQUELYN C. CAMPBELL, PhD, RN, FAAN, is the Anna D. Wolf Chair at the Johns Hopkins School of Nursing. She earned her BSN at Duke, her MSN at Wright State, and her PhD at the University of Rochester. Awards include outstanding alumnus at all three universities, three honorary doctorates, the American Society of Criminology Vollmer Award, the Institute of Medicine Senior Nurse Scholar in Residence, and the Friends of the National Institute of Nursing Research Pathfinder Award.

Dr. Campbell's specific areas of research include risk factors and assessment for intimate partner homicide; abuse during pregnancy; marital rape; physical and mental health effects of domestic violence; dating violence; and testing interventions to prevent and address domestic violence. She has authored or co-authored more than 150 articles and chapters and six books. With continuous research funding since 1984, she has been principle investigator on nine major grants from the National Institutes of Health and Justice, the Centers for Disease Control and Prevention, and the Department of Defense. She was Co-Chair of the Steering Committee for the World Health Organization Multi-Country Study of Violence Against Women and Health.

A hallmark of Dr. Campbell's career has been her collaborations with domestic violence advocacy organizations including board membership at four domestic violence shelters in Michigan, New York, and Maryland and now at the Family Violence Prevention Fund. Policy work includes the National Advisory Council on Violence Against Women, the congressionally appointed Department of Defense Task Force on Domestic Violence, former U.S. Surgeon General C. Everett Koop's Workshop on Violence and Health (1986), research agendas for CDC, NIH, and ARRQ, and three major Institute of Medicine Committees.

Assessing Dangerousness

*Violence by Batterers
and Child Abusers*

Second Edition

Jacquelyn C. Campbell, PhD, RN, FAAN
Editor

SPRINGER PUBLISHING COMPANY
NEW YORK

Springer Publishing Company, LLC
11 West 42nd Street
New York, NY 10036
www.springerpub.com

Acquisitions Editor: Jennifer Perillo
Production Editor: Carol Cain
Cover design: Joanne E. Honigman
Composition: Apex Publishing, LLC

15 16 17/ 5 4 3

Library of Congress Cataloging-in-Publication Data

Assessing dangerousness : violence by batterers and child abusers / [edited by] Jacquelyn C. Campbell. — 2nd ed.
   p. ; cm.
  Includes bibliographical references and index.
  ISBN-13: 978-0-8261-0298-0 (alk. paper)
  ISBN-10: 0-8261-0298-0 (alk. paper)
  1. Violence—Forecasting. 2. Family violence—Forecasting. 3. Sex crimes—Forecasting. I. Campbell, Jacquelyn.
  [DNLM: 1. Domestic Violence. 2. Forecasting. 3. Risk Assessment. 4. Sex Offenses. WA 308 A846 2007]
RC569.5.V55A87 2007
616.85'8200112—dc22   2007012052

Printed in the United States of America by Maple Press

Contents

About the Contributors

Carolyn Rebecca Block, PhD, is Senior Research Analyst at the Illinois Criminal Justice Information Authority. A founder of the Homicide Research Working Group, she is principal investigator of the Chicago Women's Health Risk Study, and maintains the Chicago Homicide Dataset. She is currently doing collaborative research using both of those datasets.

Nancy Glass, PhD, MPH, RN, is Associate Professor at the Johns Hopkins University School of Nursing. Her areas of interest include health disparities, intimate partner violence, and community-based participatory research methods. Dr. Glass received her BSN from the Johns Hopkins University School of Nursing, her MPH from the Johns Hopkins University Bloomberg School of Public Health, and her PhD from the University of Maryland, Baltimore.

Grant T. Harris, PhD, is Director of Research at the Mental Health Centre in Penetanguishene, Ontario. He is also adjunct Associate Professor of Psychology at Queen's University, Kingston, and adjunct Associate Professor of Psychiatry at the University of Toronto. Formerly, he was responsible for the development and supervision of behavioral programs on a maximum security unit for dangerous and assaultive men. His research interests include violent and criminal behavior, sexual aggression, psychopathy, psychopharmacology, and decision making.

N. Zoe Hilton, PhD, CPsych, is Senior Research Scientist at the Mental Health Centre in Penetanguishene, Ontario, and adjunct Assistant Professor of Psychiatry at the University of Toronto. She was formerly a forensic psychologist in the Oak Ridge maximum security facility, and conducted sex offender assessment and treatment in the Centre for Addiction and Mental Health (formerly Clarke Institute of Psychiatry) in Toronto.

Jane Koziol-McLain, PhD, RN, is an Assistant Professor and the Division Research Coordinator at the University of Auckland School of Nursing, New Zealand. She received her PhD from the University of Colorado School of Nursing and did a post doctoral fellowship at Johns Hopkins University School of Nursing. She has had four research proposals funded, and is currently funded by the New Zealand Ministry of Health to address emergency department interventions for victims of intimate partner violence. Her many publications describe important research in many aspects of domestic violence.

Richard D. Krugman, MD, is dean of the School of Medicine at the University of Colorado at Denver and Health Sciences Center and has attained international prominence in the field of child abuse. He has earned many honors in the field of child abuse and neglect, and headed the U.S. Advisory Board on Child Abuse and Neglect from 1988 to 1991. He has authored four books in addition to more than 100 original papers, chapters, and editorials. For 15 years he has served as editor-in-chief of *Child Abuse and Neglect: The International Journal.*

Scott D. Krugman, MD, is chair of the pediatrics department at Franklin Square Hospital Center, Baltimore, and faculty for the family practice residency program. In addition, he is clinical assistant professor of pediatrics at the University of Maryland School of Medicine, Baltimore. After graduating from Dartmouth Medical School (Hanover, NH), Dr. Krugman completed his pediatric residency at Johns Hopkins Hospital, Baltimore.

Barbara J. Limandri, PhD, RN, is an Associate Professor at Linfield College in Portland, Oregon. Dr. Limandri maintains a clinical and research interest in mental health of women, especially as it relates to intimate partner violence. She has 30 years experience as an educator and mental health nurse. She received her BSN from Virginia Commonwealth University, MSN from Catholic University of America and DNSc from the University of California, San Francisco.

Judith McFarlane, RN, DrPH, FAAN, is the Parry Chair in Health Promotion and Disease Prevention at Texas Woman's University, College of Nursing, in Houston, Texas. Dr. McFarlane conducts research on the health effects of violence against women and the effectiveness of interventions to prevent further violence. Her research has been funded by the National Center for Injury Prevention, Agency for Health Research & Quality, The National Institute of Justice, and the National Institutes of Health. Dr. McFarlane began studying abuse during pregnancy in 1984 and has since authored seminal studies on abuse of pregnant women and its connection with low birthweight. Her research findings have been presented to congressional committees, included in national health objectives, and used by clinicians in the U.S. and abroad to set standards of care for pregnant women.

Joel S. Milner, PhD, is professor of psychology at Northern Illinois University. His research interests are in the areas of family violence and sexual assault. Some of his research has focused on the description and explanation of child physical abuse, child sexual abuse, and adult sexual assault. Dr. Milner received his BS from the University of Houston, and his MS and PhD from Oklahoma State University.

Christine A. Poulos, BSN, RN, CHPN, is a graduate student at the Johns Hopkins University School of Nursing. She is completing her degree as a clinical nurse specialist with a focus in forensic nursing. Christine has worked as a registered nurse within hospital settings for 6 years, is currently working at Johns Hopkins Hospital and is certified in hospice and palliative care nursing. She completed her forensic nurse examiner (FNE) training in May 2006 and will graduate from Johns Hopkins in May 2008.

Daniel J. Sheridan, PhD, RN, FNE-A, FAAN, is Associate Professor at the Johns Hopkins University School of Nursing. His areas of interest include forensic nursing, domestic violence, elder abuse and neglect, abuse/neglect of vulnerable persons with disabilities, sexual assault, and child abuse and neglect. Dr. Sheridan received his PhD from Oregon Health Sciences University.

Yvonne Ulrich, PhD, RN, is retired from a productive career in nursing education and research. She received her doctorate from the University of Texas and completed a post doctoral fellowship in women's health at the University of Washington School of Nursing. She has conducted several important studies on women's experiences of domestic violence, concentrating on interpretive qualitative analysis. She continues to publish and has numerous journal articles and book chapters on women's understanding of their lives in abusive relationships.

Daniel J. Webster, MPH, ScD, is an Associate Professor and Co-Director of the Johns Hopkins Center for Gun Policy and Research in the Johns Hopkins Bloomberg School of Public Health Department of Health Policy and Management. His MPH is from the University of Michigan and ScD from Johns Hopkins University. He has an active program of research in violence prevention, and has published many articles on youth violence, intimate partner violence, evaluation of violence prevention programs and intimate partner homicide risk.

Preface

All of the contributors to this volume have been in clinical situations in which we have been asked to assess or have tried to determine how violent an individual is likely to be and how much danger his or her potential victim is actually in. In courts, clinics, conference rooms, battered women's shelters, hospital emergency rooms, child protective service offices, schools, research settings, home visits, batterer intervention programs, parenting programs, domestic violence advocacy programs, and child abuse and intimate partner violence prevention programs we have faced the difficult problem of predicting family violence just as you have and probably still do if you are interested enough in the issues to read this preface. We have been acutely aware of how this issue has profound implications, intersecting our clinical judgments, advocacy, agendas, and professional and ethical responsibilities.

The contributors are all clinicians to some extent, collaborate with practitioners from many disciplines, and share a profound respect for the work that practitioners are doing in the family violence field. But each of us has also added a research involvement to his or her clinical base. Thus we are trying to add what we know from our research to the difficult problem of clinical prediction of violence in situations of child and wife abuse and sexual violence.

We have learned a great deal over the past 20 years since the first edition of this volume, and we have tried to incorporate this information in user-friendly language and approach. We have tried to be helpful to all of us—clinicians and researchers in various combinations of history and roles—in this volume. We offer you our summary of the research in this area, as well as the instruments that may be helpful and the criteria by which to judge them. To this, you will add your own clinical expertise.

I want to first thank all the abused women who have helped me understand what it would be like to be in danger. I started this journey with a homicide study back in the late 1970s, and to all those who have been killed and their families whose lives I have marked in my research as well as all those who have died as the result of intimate partner violence and child abuse in this country and around the world, I stand in tribute and remembrance. I especially want to acknowledge Anne, whose death in 1979 inspired me to be the best clinician, advocate, and researcher I could possibly be. We must never forget the strengths of abused women like Anne. We also must not forget abused children and the incredible attempts they take every single day to keep safe and healthy.

I also would like to thank all of the contributors to this volume for their responsiveness to reviews, their patience with the process, and their collective wisdom and commitment to these issues. Especially I would like to thank Jon Conte for his leadership in creating the original volume and in the field of interpersonal violence. The staff at Springer, especially Jennifer Perillo, has been extremely helpful and patient in this production, a rather difficult process at times because of my own distractions and competing demands.

I also want to thank all of the practitioners in this field that I have trained, collaborated with, advocated with, and corresponded with over these many years. I always think of those I have known the longest: David Adams, Nancy Durborow, Ed Gondolf, Ricardo Guzman, Barbara Hart, Ann Menard, Joyce Thomas, Oliver Williams, my colleagues on the Task Force on Domestic Violence in the Military, the shelters where I have volunteered in various capacities over the years—now at the House of Ruth Maryland where Carole Alexander, Tania Araya, Dorothy Lennig, and Terri Wurmser provide such talented leadership—and last but never least, the Family Violence Prevention Fund (FVPF). I admire and am proud to work with everyone on staff at the FVPF but especially the amazing director, Esta Soler, and her leadership team, Debbie Lee, Leni Marin, and Janet Carter.

Finally, I would like to acknowledge the unfailing help and support of my students, former students, research colleagues of the Nursing Research Consortium on Violence and Abuse (each and every one of you), national and international research colleagues from all over the globe, research staff at Johns Hopkins University School of Nursing, and particular collaborators and friends in the field of family violence at Hopkins: Andrea Gielen, Nancy Glass, Joan Kub, Pate Mahoney, Phyllis Sharps, Dan Sheridan, Daniel Webster, and she who supports all of us, Nadiyah Johnson.

I would also like to extend my thanks to two moms of incredible wisdom and love, Dorothy Bowman and Constance Morrow; a father and brother committed to nonviolence, Joseph Bowman Sr. and Jr.; an incredibly brilliant sister, Deborah; an always supportive brother and sister-in-law, Patrik and Shelley; my especially wonderful children, Christy and Brad; their amazing spouses and children, Nik, Nadia, Grace, Sophie, and Nathan; and most of all to Reg, the love of my life, my thanks and love.

Jacquelyn C. Campbell, PhD, RN, FAAN
Anna D. Wolf Chair and Professor
Johns Hopkins University School of Nursing

CHAPTER 1

Prediction of Interpersonal Violence: An Introduction

Daniel J. Sheridan, Nancy Glass,
Barbara J. Limandri, and Christine A. Poulos

Clinicians who work in interpersonal violence are asked frequently to make predictions about their patients, or clients' violent behavior. Most notably, clinicians are asked by law enforcement personnel, child and elder protective services workers, and civil and criminal court officials to predict the likelihood of future violence by alleged and/or convicted family violence and sexual assault perpetrators. These assessments of "dangerousness" serve the primary functions of developing safety strategies for victims and controlling future violent behaviors of the perpetrator by treatment or confinement (Campbell & Glass, in press; Campbell, Sharps, & Glass, 2001; Gondolf, Mulvey, & Lidz, 1990).

In this chapter, we review what is generally known about the prediction of violent behavior and then discuss implications for the prediction of interpersonal violence. Succeeding chapters address the specific variables involved in the prediction of child abuse and neglect, and intimate partner violence (both heterosexual and same-sex). This volume represents the most current research, trends, and professional viewpoints regarding the prediction of interpersonal violence.

Although the prediction of interpersonal violence is a relatively young science, it is an area of utmost importance. As aptly stated by Hilton and

Harris (2005), "Predicting violence is quite a different task from explaining it" (p. 3). Clinicians working in the field will always be concerned that a case with which they have worked will end in a serious injury, homicide, or homicide-suicide unless they take every possible action to avert such an outcome. Consider the following scenario.

A CLINICAL REALITY: HOSPITAL-BASED INTERVENTION

8:00 a.m.: You are paged to the intensive care unit to see a critically injured patient just admitted from the emergency department (ED). The woman has multiple fractures to her face, bruises to her chest and back, and a partially ruptured spleen. She tells you that 2 days ago her husband struck her with a board and kicked her multiple times. He would not let her seek medical care. She thinks that earlier today she must have passed out at home from internal bleeding. She was driven to the ED by her husband, who then left the hospital. She tells you that her husband has a permit to carry a concealed weapon and that he frequently has threatened to kill her and the children if she ever tried to leave the relationship. She asks, "Will my husband beat me again? Could he kill me or my kids?"

8:25 a.m.: The hospital administrator pages you and wants to know whether this patient's husband poses a risk of harm to other patients, staff, or visitors.

8:50 a.m.: You are paged by a child protective services department investigator. She tells you she has been investigating this family because of a recent child abuse allegation filed by the school. The children did not arrive at school this morning, and they are not at home. She thinks they may be with their father. She asks you whether you think the children are at risk of abuse and whether the mother knows of their whereabouts.

9:00 a.m.: You are paged by the ED staff to see another patient, a woman who was just raped and then shot in the hip by her former husband. On the basis of the patient's initial history, the ED staff has fears that he may come to the hospital to "finish what he started." They ask whether you think this man is capable of coming to the ED to kill his former wife.

9:05 a.m.: You are paged by the prosecuting attorney's office to confirm that you will testify in court later that day around 1:00 p.m. on a case from several months ago.

PREDICTIVE SETTINGS

The above scenario is a real-life example of a day in the life of a clinician who works with domestic and sexual violence survivors in crisis. As illustrated, the clinician is called on repeatedly to make assessments and predictions of risk for repeat violence, often after obtaining only a cursory history of the violent behavior and without any direct contact with the alleged perpetrator. Clinicians in acute incident settings (e.g., hospital social workers, forensic nurses, physicians, field investigators, hot-line workers) are especially pressed for time. In these instances, predictions are likely to be best guesses, based on intuition, knowledge, experience, and often biases.

Typically this initial prediction, or assessment of risk, will be revisited several times and in a number of settings. In the criminal justice system, documentation and/or testimony regarding the defendant's propensity for violence may influence a variety of judicial outcomes. For example, the court may ask the clinician to predict the likelihood of future violence when sentencing a convicted offender. The expert opinion of the clinician may significantly affect the type and length of sentence. Likewise such testimony may influence the eligibility of convicted offenders to participate in new, innovative, deferred sentencing programs or other forms of alternative dispensation, such as community-based treatment programs. In family court, clinicians' predictions of future violence may influence the court's ruling on a protection or stalking order or on issues of child custody and protection.

Clearly the clinician's assessment of dangerousness can be an enormously valuable resource. This value highlights the need for the development of accurate and reliable models for the prediction of interpersonal violence. The accuracy of using clinical judgment to predict risk for violence has been questioned (Grove, Zald, Lebow, Snitz, & Nelson, 2000; Monohan et al., 2001). In fact, Hilton and Harris (2005), in their review of research literature predicting intimate partner violence against women, clearly state that actuarial risk assessment techniques and tools are far more accurate than unstructured clinical judgments or structured clinical risk assessment tools.

Actuarial Risk Assessment

Actuarial risk assessment is an evidence-based prediction process based on statistical analysis (Hilton & Harris, 2005). The Violence Risk Appraisal Guide (VRAG) is an actuarial risk assessment tool that was created in 1993 to address violence potential in men undergoing pretrial psychological forensic assessments (Harris, Rice, & Quinsey, 1993). It has been used to assess violence recidivism in sex offenders, prison inmates, nonforensic psychiatric patients, and domestic violence perpetrators (Hilton & Harris, 2005). While it was created to assess violence, "the VRAG may be the assessment tool of choice when measuring risk of wife assault recidivism" according to Hilton and Harris (2005), although it has not been used widely and has not been extensively validated with that population. It is composed of 12 variables that require a thorough understanding of the background of the offender and the offender's psychological adjustment, including knowledge gained from using the Hare Psychopathy Checklist-Revised (PCL-R). Thus, it takes considerable training and time to learn how to administer and evaluate findings from the VRAG (Hilton & Harris, 2005). Nonetheless, the PCL-R, developed by Hare, Clark, Grann, and Thornton (2000), is a very strong predictor of violence recidivism, in general, and specifically among more serious male abusers of women (Harris, Skilling, & Rice, 2001).

The Ontario Domestic Assault Risk Assessment (ODARA) is another actuarial risk assessment tool that contains only 13 items and was created for use by police officers in the field who respond to domestic violence emergency calls (Hilton et al., 2004). The items on the ODARA are scored 0 or 1 and include threats and confinement during the most recent assault, domestic and nondomestic criminal history, offender substance abuse, victim barriers to support, and children in the relationship (Hilton & Harris, 2005). With minimal training, police officers had perfect interrater reliability of the items on the ODARA (Hilton et al., 2004).

Does Treatment Work?

For over 20 years, court systems in North America have been ordering men into counseling in hopes of stopping or reducing their abuse toward women. The success of these programs is a matter of debate. According to Hilton and Harris (2005), "there is no scientifically persuasive evidence that current treatments for wife assaulters reduce recidivism" (p. 15). However, success of a batterer intervention program is more complex than just measuring whether the violence stopped. Gondolf (2002) found that women reported significantly less violence and improved quality of life after their partners completed batterer intervention programs and that an extremely important contributor to treatment failure was abusers dropping out of the program. Clients/patients more likely to drop out of abuser treatment tend to be younger and to have less education, less money, and unstable social lifestyles (Scott, 2004).

Craig, Browne, and Stringer (2003) reviewed the literature on sexual assault recidivism after treatment and found treatment effectiveness to be questionable. They found most promising those cognitive-behavioral treatments that targeted deviant arousal, increasing appropriate sexual desires, improving interpersonal skills, and modifying distorted thinking (Craig, Browne, & Stringer, 2003).

Veneziano and Veneziano (2002) reviewed the research on adolescent sex offenders and found they shared many characteristics that were predictive of recidivism such as: being reared in a dysfunctional home, experiencing prior physical and/or sexual abuse, separation from parents as when placed in foster care, isolation, and having academic and behavioral problems at school. Most treatment programs designed for adolescent offenders were modeled after adult offender programs, which do not have huge success rates. Not surprisingly, Veneziano and Veneziano (2002) found, in general, little research that supports any effectiveness in adolescent treatment programs. Obviously, more research is needed in treatment programs for perpetrators of many abuses in order to reduce recidivism.

CLASSIC CLINICALLY BASED PREDICTION MODELS

The prediction of interpersonal violence demands the use of psychometrically sound measurements and an understanding of such tools' limitations. Classic research in clinical decision making (Benner, 1984; Harbison, 1991; Schon, 1983a) identifies three major models for prediction: (a) the linear, rationalist model, (b) the hypothetico-deductive model, and (c) the risk assessment model (Gottfredson & Gottfredson, 1988). Depending on the goal of the assessment, the clinician may use aspects of one or more of these models.

Linear (Rationalist) Model

Because prediction has such significant forensic implications, clinicians may use a linear model, including a decision tree or critical pathway, to guide them when making decisions that have legal ramifications. For example, Gross, Southard, Lamb, and Weinberger (1987) proposed seven steps to follow when a client makes suggestive threats.

Step 1 is to clarify the threat. Many clients/patients make vague comments that may or may not indicate a real danger. Thus the clinician must take the time to fully explore intent. For example, after an acute beating, a battered woman may state that she wishes someone would "blow his [the abuser's] brains out." In this case the clinician needs to ask the client/patient directly whether she intends to kill her abuser. This woman simply may be expressing her anger rather than verbalizing a true threat. Further inquiry might reveal that she does not own or have access to a firearm. The risk factor for retaliatory violence is therefore low, especially when compared with the client/patient who tells the clinician that she would like to kill her abuser and has borrowed her brother's loaded handgun.

Thus, if there is a clear threat, Step 2 is to assess its lethality, as well as the likelihood of the person acting on the threat. As with suicidal thoughts, not all "threats" pose a true danger or can be enacted. The incarcerated client or hospitalized patient may verbalize specific threats of violence against someone outside of prison or the hospital but have no means to carry through on the threats.

If there is evidence of danger, Step 3 is to identify a specific, intended victim. In family violence and family sexual assault cases, it is easy to identify intended victims. The violence is seldom random, even within homes in which multiple members reside. The clinician working with a client/patient who is verbalizing concerns about physically and/or sexually assaulting a stranger may find it more difficult to identify a specific victim (by name). However, the clinician can ask the client/patient to indicate the intended victim's gender and any specific victim characteristics. If the person can name the intended victim or specifics about the type of victim who will be sought, the threat of harm is imminent (Step 4). At this point the clinician needs to consider his or her duty to warn the specified victim. Specifically, according to the California Supreme Court Tarasoff decision, "When a therapist determines, or pursuant to the standards of his profession should determine, that his patient presents a serious danger of violence to another, he incurs an obligation to use reasonable care to protect the intended victim against such danger. The discharge of this duty may require the therapist to take one or more of various steps. Thus, it may call for him to warn the intended victim, to notify the police, or to take whatever steps are reasonably necessary under the circumstances." For more detail the reader is referred to the body of literature on the Tarasoff decisions (*Tarasoff v. Regents of the University of California,* 1974, 1976).

The clinician also must take into account the client/patient's relationship to the intended victim (Step 5). If the intended victim is a family member, rather than a political figure, the clinician may employ different preventive and treatment strategies.

Step 6 requires the clinician to decide whether a family or couples therapy intervention would be suitable. For example, if the family violence is ongoing, family therapy may impose greater danger to the potential victim or victims.

Finally, Step 7 requires the clinician to consider whether civil commitment or involuntary hospitalization would provide the greatest good to the client/patient and potential victim or victims. At the completion of Step 7, the clinician needs to follow up on the results of the decisions made and may need to recycle through the decision tree at a later date.

The strength of the linear model is that it provides relatively clear direction for the clinician, as well as a "logical" argument for the decision. Using the linear model, the clinician approaches problem solving with some notion of probability. He or she weighs outcomes according to objective standards or theory. The weakness of this model is also its objectivity; contextually relevant information is given little consideration. In other words, factors such as treatment outcomes, social support, and stabilization of stress are not considered in making the prediction. The decision is driven by formula, more than by the specifics of the actual situation.

Hypothetico-Deductive Model

By contrast, the hypothetico-deductive model tends to be relational and complex in assessing factors that influence clinical decisions. As with the linear model, the clinician weighs different factors, but the problem is considered more in context. In addition, past experiences with similar situations provide the clinician with patterns of cues to consider and ways to categorize the cues. In considering all of the information in the current situation, the expert is searching for a "pivotal cue" to frame all of the cues and to link with extensive theoretical and experiential knowledge (Regan-Kubinski, 1991; Schon, 1983b).

After the clinician has focused his or her questioning and assessment, he or she begins to search specifically for additional cues relevant to violence and protectiveness. In clustering the cues, the expert continually loops back to the context of the specific client and to the overall context of the community in which the situation is occurring. Finally, the clinician arranges the cues into some hypotheses and reviews the hypotheses for completeness. He or she may seek additional cues to complete the picture if necessary. The hypotheses then are tested for confirmation or refutation, and a final decision is made. The following case example illustrates this process:

> While tightly clenching his fists, a young man tells his high school counselor that his grades plummeted because his girlfriend, whom he refers to in sexually derogatory terms, broke off their relationship. The counselor knows that this student has a history of frequent alcohol abuse and fighting on school grounds. The young man's father is in the Army on an extended overseas assignment in the Middle East. The mother reports that her son refuses to accept her authority and that he has become difficult to manage in the absence of the father.

Using the hypothetico-deductive model, the clinician first focuses on the cues of anger, age, rejection by the girlfriend, and alcohol abuse, reaching the pivotal cue of "potential for dangerousness." The counselor also hypothesizes that the young man may be depressed, feeling out of control, and feeling abandoned, all of which would contribute to his potential for violence. In addition, the counselor considers such cues as the school's location in New Orleans and the school's climate after Hurricane Katrina, reports of several similar situations with the other young men in the school, and reports that the girls in the school have been complaining about violence by the boys. The counselor reaches the judgment that not only is this young man potentially dangerous but also there may be a systemic problem in the school and community. Thus the immediate plan is to confront the young man's anger and to recommend some structured physical activity. The counselor also determines that the girlfriend has different classes from the boyfriend and that the possibility of contact that day is slight. The young man contracts to stay away from the girlfriend and not harm her. To meet the community problem recognized by this model, the counselor consults with his female colleague and together they plan a special assembly on the topic of dating violence. They also set up gender-segregated peer groups to discuss violence in the community and within dating relationships.

Risk Assessment Model

A major reason for poor predictive accuracy of interpersonal violence is the assumption that violence is dichotomous and single dimensional (Gottfredson & Gottfredson, 1988). Instead of a binary notion of violence, Gottfredson and Gottfredson propose a risk-to-stakes matrix wherein the seriousness of the action is weighed with the likelihood of repetition. Seriousness permits the assessor to consider types of harm possible across a multitude of variables.

Alcohol and drug use, for example, might influence the likelihood of harm, as well might a history of violence. By means of the risk assessment model, clinicians can provide assessments of risk factors or risk markers that may contribute to violence. Such a model incorporates the social and political climate, as well as the individual's internal climate. The risk assessment model permits clinicians to weigh both the environmental and personal factors present in any given situation. The following case demonstrates this model:

> Convicted of felony assault on his former girlfriend, a 28-year-old male with a history of alcoholism is up for parole after serving half of a 12-month sentence. While in prison, he completed extensive alcohol treatment and anger management programs. On release from jail he intends to live with his mother. As the clinician, it would be imperative to know that his mother lives less than a block from the former girlfriend and that living in the mother's home are several alcoholic siblings. Releasing this man into his mother's home, into close contact with alcoholic siblings, places him at high risk for drinking. Because his mother lives so close to his former girlfriend, further abuse and stalking is also quite possible. Instead of recommending against parole, the clinician may advise that parole be contingent on housing arrangements that do not place the offender in such close contact with either alcohol or his prior victim.

The three clinical decision-making models discussed above are distinct, but not necessarily exclusive, means for deciding on interventions. In courtrooms, linear decision routes are much easier to substantiate. However, decisions are rarely so clear-cut in the clinical arena. Therefore, clinicians need to be adept in approaching (or at least justifying) these decisions from multiple perspectives.

PREDICTIVE RELIABILITY AND VALIDITY

The accuracy (validity) and consistency (reliability) of predicting dangerousness and violence depends on multiple, complex factors. In general, the more rare an event, the more difficult it is to predict (Campbell, Webster, & Glass, in press; Lambert, Cartor, & Walker, 1988; Webster et al., 2003). For example, predicting the risk of intimate partner violence (IPV) re-assault has become the primary aim of the majority of IPV risk assessment instruments. IPV re-assault is easier to accurately predict because it has a much higher occurrence (approximately 25% to 30% of IPV cases) than does intimate partner homicide (approximately .04% of IPV cases) (Campbell, 2004).

Factors that are known to influence the accuracy, or validity, of predicting dangerousness include: the type of violence (e.g., physical assault, sexual assault, homicide); the perpetrator's relationship to the victim (e.g., stranger, intimate, acquaintance); the characteristics of the perpetrators (e.g., history of violence, mental health issues); and the time period of the prediction (e.g., acute danger or chronic danger).

The succeeding chapters discuss in greater depth challenges with assessment measures and factors used to predict future violence. It is clear, however, that assessments of risk for future violence are improved when appropriately administered, psychometrically sound risk assessment scales are used. Further, clinicians need to couple these objective measures with information collected on the characteristics of the perpetrators, the perpetrator's relationship to victim, the victim's assessment of risk, clinician experience and judgment, and context-specific factors (e.g., poverty, unemployment, discrimination, social support).

Poor Record of Past Predictions

Clinicians, in general, have a poor track record of predicting future violence among perpetrators of violence (Convit, Jaeger, Lin, Meisner, & Volavka, 1988; Gondolf et al., 1990; McNeil, Binder, & Greenfield, 1988; Miller & Morris, 1988). For example, although an assessment of danger to others and/or self is a basic assessment element of involuntary confinement or psychiatric treatment, individual clinicians have not been very successful in accurately predicting this danger for violence victims (Beigel, Barren, & Harding, 1984; McNeil et al., 1988; Meloy, 1987; Steadman & Morrissey, 1982).

However, when clinicians consult with each other (e.g., multidisciplinary review boards) and with victims of violence, they are able to pool their diverse knowledge and expertise in reaching a consensus. The social worker, psychologist, advanced nurse clinician, psychiatrist, counselor, parole officer, and victim have very different perspectives; together they form a more complete assessment of risk for future violence.

We also are learning that predictions can be made more accurately when evaluators take into account such interactive factors as age, gender, unemployment, perpetrator-victim relationship status, perpetrator's history of violence, use of alcohol and/or illegal substances, history of mental health issues, and availability of guns (Campbell et al., 2001; Meloy, 1987; Segal, Watson, Goldfinger, & Averbuck, 1988). Although risk factors such as age, gender, and prior history of violence cannot be changed by intervention, risk factors such as unemployment, perpetrator access to gun, and use of alcohol and illegal drugs can be the focus of intervention. Risk for future violence may thereby be reduced (Campbell et al., 2003).

PREDICTIVE FACTORS

History of Violence

Research into the prediction of interpersonal violence consistently shows that a history of violence is one of the best predictors of future violence (Convit et al., 1988; Janofsky, Spears, & Neubauer, 1988; Lewis, Lovely, Yeager, & Femina, 1989; McNeil et al., 1988). For example, the most important risk factor of homicide in an intimate relationship is violence against the female partner. Approximately 67%–75% of intimate partner homicides have a reported history of IPV against the female partner, no matter which partner is killed (Bailey et al., 1997; Campbell, 1992; Campbell et al., 2003; McFarlane, Parker, Soeken, Silva, & Reed, 1999; Mercy et al., 1989; Moracco, Runyan, & Butts, 1998; Pataki, 1997; Websdale, 1999).

Two studies in different U.S. jurisdictions (Dayton, Ohio, and the state of North Carolina) documented that intimate partner homicides against men were characterized by a documented history of violence against the female perpetrator by the male partner or ex-partner victim in as many as 75% of the cases (Campbell, 1992; Hall-Smith, Moracco, & Butts, 1998; Moracco et al., 1998).

When predicting reoccurrence of intimate partner violence, one important source of information about the likelihood of re-assault is the victim (Hilton et al., 2004; Weisz, Tolman, & Saunders, 2000). "Battered women's rated likelihood of partner violence strongly correlated with violence in subsequent months and years, over and above history, and other predictors" (Hilton & Harris, 2005, p. 7). However, psychometrically validated instruments were somewhat more accurate than victim perception in an experimental test of IPV risk assessment (Campbell, O'Sullivan, Roehl, & Webster, 2005).

There is limited research on risk factors for lethal or near-lethal violence in marginalized populations such as sexual minorities. For example, data from the Supplemental Homicide Reports (SHR) estimate that from 1981 to 1998, 6.2% of the total murder rate for men in the United States was male same-sex couple intimate partner homicides in comparison to 0.5% female same-sex partners homicides. However, we have been unable to find any systematic study of risk factors for male same-sex partner homicides, and there has been only one study of female same-sex intimate partner homicides (Glass, Koziol-McLain, Campbell, & Block, 2004). In that subsample analysis of five intimate partner homicides and four attempted intimate partner homicides by female partners, a prior history of violence by the female intimate partner was a notable risk factor to the lethal or near-lethal violence event.

Although a history of violence is a risk factor consistent with lethal and near-lethal violence in heterosexual couples, because of the small sample, definitive conclusions cannot be drawn for risk factors in female same-sex relationships. Currently, Glass and colleagues are conducting a study to better understand and assess for risk factors for repeat violence in abusive female same-sex relationships.

Mental Illness

Further research is needed to explicate the link between mental illness and risk for violence and repeat violence. Studies have produced mixed information regarding the role of mental health issues and violence perpetration. Given information for one study, perpetrators of intimate partner homicide appear to be more likely to have a history of mental illness. Specifically, 13% of perpetrators (11% of males, 15% of females) of 540 intimate partner homicides had a reported history of mental illness, that is compared to 3% (not reported by gender) of nonfamily murderers (Zawitz, 1994).

In other data, approximately one-third of the 200 male perpetrators from a multicity study of lethal and near-lethal intimate partner violence were described as being in poor (versus fair, good, or excellent) mental health (Sharps, Campbell, Campbell, Gary, & Webster, 2001). Although perpetrator mental health was significantly associated to risk for intimate partner homicide, it did not remain significant when examined with other factors in the multivariate analysis for the study (Sharps et al., 2001). In the Dobash et al. (2004) United Kingdom study, 27.5% of the men who perpetrated intimate partner homicide were labeled as having mental health problems, a proportion approximately the same as men who perpetrated other types of murder (non–intimate partner).

Perpetrators who are psychopaths have a high likelihood of re-offending. While psychopaths represent a relatively small percentage of men who abuse women (15% to 30%) their behavioral traits of superficial charm, need for stimulation, callousness, and manipulation are quite familiar to clinicians who provide service to their victims (Hilton & Harris, 2005). Psychopaths will have a history of early behavioral problems, impulsivity, antisocial behavior, and callousness.

Clinicians are often called upon to make predictions of dangerousness as a requirement of their roles in health care settings such as psychiatric hospitals and emergency departments, but as mentioned earlier, clinicians are often not provided with the training related to assessment of dangerousness and, therefore, have historically had a poor rate of predictive accuracy (Quinsey, Harris Rice & Cormier, 2006). Because of (or in spite of) these poor predictive accuracy rates, there is great internal and external pressure on clinicians to develop more effective means of identifying patients or clients who are likely to be violent.

One challenge to assessing risk of violence among patients or clients who have been diagnosed with a mental illness is the criteria used to identify "violent" acts and "violent" people. For example, psychiatric patients or clients have traditionally been assessed for danger to self and danger to others. As a result, suicide and self-mutilation may be included in the findings, potentially overestimating the patient's or client's dangerousness. Likewise, the patient or client may demonstrate very different patterns of behavior when hospitalized (Holcomb & Ahr, 1988; Myers & Dunner, 1984) simply because they are receiving treatment. Because the severe mental illnesses (e.g., schizophrenia, bipolar disorder) are relapsing ones, violence is a greater factor in times of decompensation and psychosis than during stabilization (Craig, 1982; Krakowski, Jaeger, & Volavka, 1988; Tardiff & Sweillman, 1982).

Substance Abuse

Although alcohol and/or drug abuse has classically been frequently reported as the cause of interpersonal violence, most research describes a relationship between the use of alcohol and other substances with incidents of violence (Dobash & Dobash, 1979; Frieze & Schafer, 1984; Goodman, Mercy, & Loya, 1986; Goodman, Mercy, & Rosenberg, 1986; Lenke, 1982; Norton & Morgan, 1989a, 1989b, 1989c).

Alcohol

The majority of research articles on substance use and its relationship to violence focus on alcohol usage, mainly of the perpetrator. To understand this potential causal relationship, it is important to understand the effects of alcohol on the body. Alcohol is a depressant, with its short-acting action associated with arousing, euphoric effects followed by dysphoric, depressing effects. Its effect on behavior can be roughly correlated with the level of alcohol present in the body as measured by blood alcohol content, although it does not follow a simple pharmacologic dose-effect relationship, and is different in each person (Miczek et al., 1994).

Theoretical explanations of alcohol's role in child and partner violence consider both proximal and distal influences. The proximal effect model is that there should be a temporal relationship between substance use and violence, meaning that episodes of violent acts would closely follow ingestion of the substance. The psychopharmacologic effects of alcohol on cognitive processing facilitate violent behavior, in that persons having ingested significant amounts of alcohol are more likely to interpret others' behavior as hostile and are less likely to be able to problem solve a nonviolent solution to conflict, especially if they have learned violent behaviors in their family of origin. Distal influences include individual difference factors such as personality characteristics and life experiences and contextual influences such as relationship type, all of which may create an environment that facilitates violent behavior, especially when added to alcohol (Chermack & Blow, 2002; Fals-Stewart, Golden, & Schumacher, 2003). Regardless of the theories, alcohol use is one of the accepted risk factors for child and partner violence.

Fals-Stewart (2003) discovered in his longitudinal diary study that the likelihood of male-to-female aggression was substantially higher on days of drinking by male partners compared with days of no drinking. In fact, physical aggression was 8–11 times higher on days of drinking. Also, it was determined that the violence occurred shortly after the drinking episodes ended, supporting the proximal effects model described above. The study concluded "use of alcohol by the male partner is a significant risk factor for the occurrence of physical aggression among couples with a history of interpartner violence" (Fals-Stewart, 2003, p. 50).

Additionally, Fals-Stewart et al. (2003) studied male-to-female physical aggression over a 15-month period to determine that interpersonal violence was significantly higher on days of alcohol use. Once again, there was a decelerating relationship between the amount of time between cessation of use and the occurrence of violence, supporting the proximal role of substance use in occurrences of IPV.

Alcohol use was significantly higher on days where physical violence and interpersonal conflict occurred, and alcohol consumption appeared to be the most potent predictor (Chermack & Blow, 2002; Thompson & Kingree, 2004). Although alcohol use is an accepted risk factor for IPV, there still remains controversy on whether there is enough evidence-based practice to support this assumption (Gil-Gonzalez, Vives-Cases, Alvarez-Dardet, & Latour-Perez, 2006). "The marked correlations between alcoholism and various types of violent acts do not permit, however, any clear insight into the pharmacologic conditions of alcohol exposure that are necessary or sufficient for these violence-promoting effects" (Miczek et al., 1994).

Other Substances

Cocaine

Cocaine is a central nervous system stimulant, the strongest stimulant derived from natural sources. Initially, use of this drug reduces appetite and makes the user feel more alert, energetic, and euphoric. With high doses, users can become delusional, paranoid, and even suffer acute toxic psychosis. As the drug's effects wear off, depression sets in, leaving the user feeling fatigued and anxious. Cocaine has also been shown to increase the incidence of IPV (Chermack & Blow, 2002; Fals-Stewart et al., 2003). It is important to also recognize the correlation of alcohol and cocaine; the interaction between the two drugs could account for the resulting effects related to aggression.

Methamphetamine

Methamphetamine is an intense, man-made stimulant. Upon ingestion, it releases high levels of the neurotransmitter dopamine, which causes excitation, euphoria, intensification of emotions, increased alertness, and heightened sexuality. Unlike other stimulants, methamphetamine is metabolized at a slower rate. Because of this, a sustained euphoric state is produced that can last up to 8 hours (Cartier, Farabee, & Prendergast, 2006). A 2006 survey of United States counties found that more counties (48%) report methamphetamine as the primary drug problem than cocaine, marijuana, and heroin combined. Additionally, 62% of counties reported an increase in domestic violence and a 53% increase in simple assaults between 2004 and 2005 (National Association of Counties, 2005).

Despite the overwhelming prevalence of methamphetamine use, there is a paucity of research examining use of the drug related to IPV. Von Mayrhauser, Brecht, and Anglin (2002) found that about two-thirds of methamphetamine users studied reported violent behavior as a result of their usage. In a multi-state study from 1999 to 2001, 1,016 methamphetamine users were examined. Eighty percent of women participating in the study reported abuse or violence by a partner (Cohen et al., 2003). It is difficult to assess from this data how much contribution methamphetamine makes to the pattern of violence reported. Researchers need to evaluate the use of methamphetamine and IPV more. Because of the heightened sexuality that the drug stimulates, researchers also need to examine possible correlation with sexual violence as well.

An important barrier exists in examining the relationship between substance abuse and violence: It is difficult to identify with certainty a perpetrator's substance abuse at the time of a violent incident. If the perpetrator has committed suicide or has volunteered samples at the time of the incident, then blood alcohol and other toxin levels are available to evaluate substance abuse potential.

Recent research has examined the role of alcohol and substance use in interpersonal violence. For example, perpetrator problem drinking and illicit drug use were significantly related to lethal violence in intimate relationships in the multicity study examining risk factors for intimate partner homicide (Campbell et al., 2003). However, neither perpetrator problem drinking nor perpetrator illicit drug use prior to the violent event were significant predictors of lethal violence when controlling for other important factors, such as use of a gun, threats to kill, and a nonbiological child of the perpetrator in the home.

Illicit drug use was a stronger predictor of lethal violence in the study than problem drinking and it did remain as a significant predictor of lethal violence until perpetrator aggressive behavior toward the partner was added into the risk model. Although subsumed by more powerful predictors (especially gun use) at the incident level, a remarkable 70% of the male perpetrators were using drugs and/or alcohol at the time of the homicidal incident (Campbell et al., 2003; Sharps, Campbell, Campbell, Gary, & Webster, 2003). Dobash et al. (2004) found that although a substantial proportion of intimate partner perpetrators had alcohol and drug problems (37.9% and 14.7% respectively), alcohol and drug problems were reported in a significantly higher proportion of males who commit other types of murders (nonintimate murder).

Gender

The literature about interpersonal violence tends to be gender-specific, depending on discussions about perpetrators or about victims. For example, many of the studies seeking to identify factors related to delinquency and violence have looked only at male behaviors (Josephson, 1987; Lewis et al., 1989; Mulvey & Reppucci, 1988). Therefore, the research provides a limited perspective on the precursors to interpersonal violence perpetrated by females. In the case of intimate partner violence, research indicates that women are more likely to report violence by an intimate partner that resulted in an injury (Tjaden & Thoennes, 2000).

Research on the effects of childhood exposure to violence, including witnessing violence, on later aggression is inconclusive. In their review of police records, Lewis et al. (1989) found that juvenile violence was not sufficient explanation for violent criminal behavior as an adult. Instead they found it to be an interaction between a history of abuse and/or family violence and the cognitive, psychiatric, and neurological impairments of the child.

Race/Ethnicity

There are clear racial/ethnic disparities in rates of intimate partner homicide, with Native American and African American women at increased risk (Mercy & Saltzman, 1989; Morton, Runyan, Moracco, & Butts, 1998). Although a significant proportion of this variation can be explained by increased rates of unemployment among Native American and African American men (Campbell et al., 2003), few investigations have tried to delineate what accounts for these discrepancies. In the 11-city study, although the majority of risk factors were similar for the African American, White, Hispanic, and mixed-race couples, we found different strengths of risk factors in certain groups and some risk factors not applying for some groups (Walton-Moss, Campbell, & Sharps, in press).

For instance, prior arrest was found to be strongly protective against intimate partner homicide for White and mixed-race couples but not protective at all for African American and Hispanic couples. When looking at the data more closely, this was related to the finding that males in ethnic minority groups who killed their partners were more frequently arrested than the White male killers, and those ethnic minority men were equally often arrested among both the lethal and abusive control groups.

ETHICAL CONSIDERATIONS

Although the empirical study of the prediction of interpersonal violence is important, a number of moral and ethical issues should be considered. The clinician who must render an assessment of the probability of future violence has a responsibility to weigh several ethical issues; he or she must consider not only the social injustice of violence perpetrated against the victim but must also weigh the perpetrator's individual rights to autonomy and freedom.

An ethical concern for clinicians is using mental health interventions as a form of social control of violent behavior versus using them to alleviate emotional and psychological distress potentially linked to violent behavior. In other words, when the clinician recommends commitment of an individual judged to be "dangerous," is the purpose of the action to help or control the perpetrator? If social control is the purpose, what treatment is ethical and appropriate—psychotropic medications or psychotherapy? Is informed consent necessary for the provision of treatment and is such consent even possible within a coercive environment?

Another problematic issue regarding the prediction of interpersonal violence is the potential for racism and classism. Evidence indicates that people of color are more likely to be prosecuted and convicted of violent crimes than white people (Spohn, 2000). Race, ethnicity, and class influence clinical judgment, as every clinician can be influenced by his or her identification with the victim or the offender.

Whether or not we participate in formal research to test the predictive properties of a particular instrument or assessment method, all clinicians make predictions about dangerousness. It can be argued that it is not possible to truly refrain from making "predictions." These predictions may be based on such factors as past behaviors, risk factors, similar behaviors that have been observed in others, clinical evaluation of the alleged offender, conversation with the victim, and/or risk assessment instruments.

Some clinicians will tend to under-predict (false negative—the person is predicted to be less dangerous than he or she actually is) the potential for danger, while others may over-predict (false positive—the person is predicted to be more dangerous than he or she actually is). If they under-predict the risk of further violence, the clinicians place the potential victim at risk of being killed or seriously hurt. When the clinician over-predicts the potential for danger, the potential victim may lose trust in the clinician's ability to identify dangerous perpetrators and situations. The client may choose to ignore future assessments by the clinician, again being placed in a vulnerable position. To over-predict the potential dangerousness of an identified perpetrator also may be to participate in a process that unjustly incarcerates, labels, and/or blames a person for past behaviors. The difficult task for the clinician is to make a judgment between the two extremes. Obviously, this requires training, skill, and a willingness to weight multiple factors using validated measures as well as trusting the opinions of colleagues and the victim(s) (Campbell, Webster, & Glass, publication submitted for review).

SUMMARY

In general, there is a series of behaviors that should raise concerns that violence will re-occur in any number of settings. These behaviors include the following:

- Prior history of being violent
- Experiencing violence as a child
- Substance abuse
- History of mental illness, especially psychopathy and antisocial behaviors
- Failing to complete an offender treatment program
- Being young and poor
- Unemployment

In intimate partner relationships all of the above are risk factors for violence with the addition of the following as risk factors for women in heterosexual relationships:

- Leaving an abusive relationship for another man
- Having a child or children from a previous relationship
- Stalking
- His access to firearms

Assessing dangerousness for further violence by sexual offenders, batterers, and child abusers is a developing science. The following chapters explore the most current research, trends, and professional viewpoints regarding the prediction of interpersonal violence.

REFERENCES

Bailey, J. E., Kellerman, A. L., Somes, G. W., Banton, J. G., Rivara, F. P., & Rushford, N. P. (1997). Risk factors for violent death of women in the home. *Archives of Internal Medicine, 157,* 777–782.

Beigel, A., Barren, M. R., & Harding, T. W. (1984). The paradoxical impact of a commitment statute on prediction of dangerousness. *American Journal of Psychiatry, 341*(3), 373–377.

Benner, P. (1984). *From novice to expert: Excellence and power in clinical nursing practice.* Reading, MA: Addison-Wesley.

Campbell, J. C. (1992). "If I can't have you, no one can": Power and control in homicide of female partners. In J. Radford & D. E. H. Russell (Eds.), *Femicide: The politics of woman killing* (pp. 99–113). New York: Twayne.

Campbell, J. C. (2004). Helping women understand their risk in situations of intimate partner violence. *Journal of Interpersonal Violence, 19*(12), 1464–1477.

Campbell, J. C., & Glass, N. (in press). Safety planning, danger, and lethality assessment. In C. Mitchell (Ed.), *Health care response to domestic violence*. Oxford University Press.

Campbell, J. C., O'Sullivan, C., Roehl, J., & Webster, D. W. (2005). Intimate partner violence risk assessment validation study: The RAVE study. Final report to the National Institute of Justice. (NCJ 209731–209732). Retrieved January 8, 2007, from http://www.ncjrs.org/pdffiles1/nij/grants/209731.pdf

Campbell, J. C., Sharps, P., & Glass, N. (2001). Risk assessment for intimate partner violence. In G. F. Pinard & L. Pagani (Eds.), *Clinical assessment of dangerousness: Empirical contributions*. New York: Cambridge University Press.

Campbell, J. C., Webster, D., & Glass, N. E. (in press). The danger assessment: Validation of a lethality risk assessment instrument for intimate partner femicide. *Journal of Interpersonal Violence.*

Campbell, J. C., Webster, D., Koziol-McLain, J., Block, C. R., Campbell, D. W., Curry, M. A., et al. (2003). Risk factors for femicide in abusive relationships: Results from a multisite case control study. *American Journal of Public Health, 93*(7), 1089–1097.

Cartier, J., Farabee, D., & Prendergast, M. L. (2006). Methamphetamine use, self-reported crime, and recidivism among offenders in California who abuse substances. *Journal of Interpersonal Violence, 21*(4), 435–445.

Chermack, S. T., & Blow, F. C. (2002). Violence among individuals in substance abuse treatment: The role of alcohol and cocaine consumption. *Drug and Alcohol Dependence, 66,* 29–37.

Cohen, J. B., Dickow, A., Horner, K., Zweben, J. E., Balabis, J., Vandersloot, D., et al. (2003). Abuse and violence: History of men and women in treatment for methamphetamine dependence. *The American Journal on Addictions, 12,* 377–385.

Convit, A., Jaeger, J., Lin, S. P., Meisner, M., & Volavka, J. (1988). Predicting assaultiveness in psychiatric inpatients: A pilot study. *Hospital and Community Psychiatry, 39*(4), 429–434.

Craig, L. A., Browne, K. D., & Stringer, I. (2003). Risk scales and factors predictive of sexual offense recidivism. *Trauma, Violence, & Abuse, 4*(1), 45–69.

Craig, T. J. (1982). An epidemiological study of problems associated with violence among psychiatric inpatients. *American Journal of Psychiatry, 139,* 1262–1266.

Dobash, R. E., & Dobash, R. (1979). *Violence against wives*. New York: Free Press.

Dobash, R. E., Dobash, R. P., Cavanagh, K., & Lewis, R. (2004). Not an ordinary killer—just an ordinary guy. When men murder an intimate woman partner. *Violence Against Women, 10,* 577–605.

Fals-Stewart, W. (2003). The occurrence of partner physical aggression on days of alcohol consumption: A longitudinal diary study. *Journal of Consulting and Clinical Psychology, 71*(1), 41–52.

Fals-Stewart, W., Golden, J., & Schumacher, J. A. (2003). Intimate partner violence and substance use: A longitudinal day-to-day examination. *Addictive Behaviors, 38,* 1555–1574.

Frieze, I. H., & Schafer, P. C. (1984). Alcohol use and marital violence: Female and male differences in reactions to alcohol. In S. C. Wilsnack & L. J. Beckrnan (Eds.), *Alcohol problems in women: Antecedents, consequences, and intervention* (pp. 260–279). New York: Guilford.

Gil-Gonzalez, D., Vives-Cases, C., Alvarez-Dardet, C., & Latour-Perez, J. (2006). Alcohol and intimate partner violence: Do we have enough information to act? *European Journal of Public Health, 16*(3), 278–284.

Glass, N. E., Koziol-McLain, J., Campbell, J. C., & Block, C. R. (2004). Female-perpetrated femicide and attempted femicide. *Violence Against Women, 10,* 606–625.

Gondolf, E. W. (2002). *Batterer intervention systems. Issues, outcomes, and recommendations.* Thousand Oaks, CA: Sage Publication.

Gondolf, E. W., Mulvey, E. P., & Lidz, C. W. (1990). Characteristics of perpetrators of family and non-family assaults. *Hospital and Community Psychiatry, 41*(2), 191–193.

Goodman, R. A., Mercy, J. A., & Loya, F. (1986). Alcohol use and interpersonal violence: Alcohol detected in homicide victims. *American Journal of Public Health, 76,* 144–146.

Goodman, R. A., Mercy, J. A., & Rosenberg, M. L. (1986). Drug use and interpersonal violence. *American Journal of Epidemiology, 124*(5), 851–855.

Gottfredson, D. M., & Gottfredson, S. D. (1988). Stakes and risks in the prediction of violent criminal behavior. *Violence and Victims, 3*(4), 247–262.

Gross, B. H., Southard, M. J., Lamb, R., & Weinberger, L. E. (1987). Assessing dangerousness and responding appropriately: *Hedlund* expands the clinician's liability established by *Tarasoff. Journal of Clinical Psychiatry, 48*(1), 9–12.

Grove, W. M., Zald, D. H., Lebow, B. S., Snitz, B. E., & Nelson, C. (2000). Clinical versus mechanical prediction: A meta-analysis. *Psychological Assessment, 12,* 19–30.

Hall-Smith, P., Moracco, K. E., & Butts, J. (1998). Partner homicide in context. *Homicide Studies, 2*(4), 400–421.

Harbison, J. (1991). Clinical decision making in nursing. *Journal of Advanced Nursing, 16,* 404–407.

Hare, R. D., Clark, D., Grann, M., & Thornton, D. (2000). Psychopathy and the predictive validity of the PCL-R: An international perspective. *Behavioral Sciences & the Law. 18*(5), 623–645.

Harris, G. T., Rice, M. E., & Quinsey, V. L. (1993). Violent recidivism of mentally disordered offenders: The development of a statistical prediction instrument. *Criminal Justice and Behavior, 20,* 315–335.

Harris, G. T., Skilling, T. A., & Rice, M. E. (2001). The construct of psychopathy. In M. Tonry (Ed.), *Criminal justice: An annual review of research* (pp. 197–294). Chicago: University of Chicago Press.

Heckert, D. A., & Gondolf, E. W. (2004). Battered women's perceptions of risk versus risk factors and instruments in predicting repeat reassault. *Journal of Interpersonal Violence, 19*(7), 778–800.

Hilton, N. Z, & Harris, G. T., (2005). Predicting wife assault: A critical review and implications for policy and practice. *Trauma, Violence, & Abuse, 6*(1), 3–23.

Hilton, N. Z., Harris, G. T., Rice, M. E., Lang, C., Cormier, C. A., & Lines, K. (2004). A brief accurate actuarial assessment for the prediction of wife assault recidivism: The Ontario Domestic Assault Risk Assessment. *Psychological Assessment, 16,* 300–312.

Holcomb, W. R., & Ahr, P. R. (1988). Arrest rates among young adult psychiatric patients treated in inpatient and outpatient settings. *Hospital and Community Psychiatry, 39,* 52–57.

Janofsky, J. S., Spears, S., & Neubauer, D. N. (1988). Psychiatrists' accuracy in predicting violent behavior on an inpatient unit. *Hospital and Community Psychiatry, 39,* 1090–1094.

Josephson, W. L. (1987). Television violence and children's aggression: Testing the priming, social script, and disinhibition predictions. *Journal of Personality and Social Psychology, 53*(5), 882–890.

Krakowski, M., Jaeger, J., & Volavka, J. (1988). Violence and psychopathology: A longitudinal study. *Comprehensive Psychiatry, 29,* 174–181.

Lambert, E. W., Cartor, R., & Walker, G. L. (1988). Reliability of behavioral versus medical models: Rare events and danger. *Issues in Mental Health Nursing, 9,* 31–44.

Lenke, L. (1982). Alcohol and crimes of violence: A causal analysis. *Contemporary Drug Problems, 11,* 355–365.

Lewis, D. O., Lovely, R., Yeager, C., & Femina, D. D. (1989). Toward a theory of the genesis of violence: A follow-up study of delinquents. *Journal of the American Academy of Child and Adolescent Psychiatry, 28*(3), 431–436.

McFarlane, J., Parker, B., Soeken, K., Silva, C., & Reed, S. (1999). Severity of abuse before and during pregnancy for African American, Hispanic, and Anglo women. *Journal of Nurse-Midwifery, 44*(2), 139–144.

McNeil, D. E., Binder, R. L., & Greenfield, T. K. (1988). Predictors of violence in civilly committed acute psychiatric patients. *American Journal of Psychiatry, 145*(8), 965–970.

Meloy, J. R. (1987). The prediction of violence in outpatient psychotherapy. *American Journal of Psychotherapy, 61*(1), 38–45.

Mercy, J. A., & Saltzman, L. E. (1989). Fatal violence among spouses in the United States 1976–85. *American Journal of Public Health, 79,* 595–599.

Miczek, K., Debold, J., Haney, M., Tidey, J., Vivian, J., & Weerts, E. (1994). Understanding and preventing violence. In A. J. Reiss, Jr. & J. A. Roth (Eds.), *Panel on the understanding and control of violent behavior* (Vol. 3, pp. 377–570). Washington, DC: National Academy Press.

Miller, M., & Morris, N. (1988). Predictions of dangerousness: An argument for limited use. *Violence and Victims, 3*(4), 263–283.

Monahan, J., Steadman, H., Silver, E., Applebaum, A., Robbins, P., Mulvey, E., et al. (2001). *Rethinking risk assessment: The Macarthur study of mental disorder and violence.* New York: Oxford University Press.

Moracco, K. E., Runyan, C. W., & Butts, J. (1998). Femicide in North Carolina. *Homicide Studies, 2,* 422–446.

Morton, E., Runyan, C. W., Moracco, K. E., & Butts, J. (1998). Partner homicide victims: A population based study in North Carolina, 1988–1992. *Violence and Victims, 13*(2), 91–106.

Mulvey, E. P., & Reppucci, N. D. (1988). The context of clinical judgment: The effect of resource availability on judgments of amenability to treatment in juvenile offenders. *American Journal of Community Psychology, 16*(4), 525–545.

Myers, K. M., & Dunner, D. L. (1984). Self- and other-directed violence on a closed acute-care ward. *Psychiatric Quarterly, 56,* 178–188.

National Association of Counties. (2005). *The meth epidemic in America: The criminal effect of meth on communities. A 2005 survey on U.S. counties.* Retrieved January 7, 2007, from http://www.naco.org/Content/ContentGroups/Publications1/Surveys1/Special_Surveys/MethSurveys.pdf

Norton, R. N., & Morgan, M. Y. (1989a). Improving information on the role of alcohol in interpersonal violence in Great Britain. *Alcohol and Alcoholism, 24*(6), 577–589.

Norton, R. N., & Morgan, M. Y. (1989b). Mortality from interpersonal violence in Great Britain. *Injury, 20,* 131–133.

Norton, R. N., & Morgan, M. Y. (1989c). The role of alcohol in mortality and morbidity from interpersonal violence. *Alcohol and Alcoholism, 24*(6), 565–576.

Pataki, G. (1997). *Intimate partner homicides in New York state.* Albany, NY: NY.

Quinsey, V. L., Harris, G. T., Rice, M. E., & Cormier, C. A. (2006). *Violent offenders: Appraising and managing risk,* 2nd Ed., Washington, DC: American Psychological Association.

Regan-Kubinski, M. J. (1991). A model of clinical judgment processes in psychiatric nursing. *Archives of Psychiatric Nursing, 5*(5), 262–270.

Schon, D. (1983a). *The reflective practitioner.* New York: Basic Books.

Schon, D. (1983b). From technical rationality to reflection in action. In J. Dowie & A. Elstein (Eds.), *Professional judgment: A reader in clinical decision making* (pp. 60–77). Cambridge, UK: Cambridge University Press.

Scott, K. L. (2004). Predictors of change among male batterers: Application of theories and review of empirical findings. *Trauma, Violence, & Abuse, 5*(3), 260–284.

Segal, S. P., Watson, M. A., Goldfinger, S. M., & Averbuck, D. S. (1988). Civil commitment in the psychiatric emergency room: The assessment of dangerousness by emergency room clinicians. *Archives of General Psychiatry, 45,* 748–752.

Sharps, P. W., Campbell, J. C., Campbell, D. W., Gary, F. A., & Webster, D. W. (2001). The role of alcohol use in intimate partner femicide. *The American Journal on Addictions, 10,* 122–135.

Sharps, P. W., Campbell, J. C., Campbell, D. W., Gary, F. A., & Webster, D. W. (2003). Risky mix: Drinking, drug use, and homicide. *NIJ Journal, 250,* 8–13.

Spohn, C. (2000). Thirty-years of sentencing reform: The quest for a racially neutral sentencing process. *Criminal Justice, 3,* National Institute of Justice.

Steadman, H. J., & Morrissey, J. P. (1982). Predicting violent behavior: A note on a cross-validation study. *Social Forces, 61,* 475–483.

Tarasoff v. Regents of the University of California. 118 Cal Rptr, 129, 529 P.2d 553 (1974).

Tarasoff v. Regents of the University of California. 17 Cal 3d 425; 551 P.2d 334 (1976).

Tardiff, K., & Sweillman, A. (1982). Assaultive behavior among chronic inpatients. *American Journal of Psychiatry, 139,* 212–215.

Thompson, M. P., & Kingree, J. B. (2004). The role of alcohol use in intimate partner violence and non-intimate partner violence. *Violence and Victims, 19*(1), 63–74.

Tjaden, P., & Thoennes, N. (2000). *Full report of the prevalence, incidence, and consequences of violence against women* (Rep. No. NCJ 183781). Washington, DC: U.S. Department of Justice, Office of Justice Programs.

Veneziano, C., & Veneziano, L. (2002). Adolescent sex offenders: A review of the literature. *Trauma, Violence, & Abuse, 3*(4), 247–260.

Von Mayrhauser, C., Brecht, M., & Anglin, M. D. (2002). Use ecology and drug use motivation of methamphetamine users admitted to substance abuse treatment facilities in Los Angeles: An emerging profile. *Journal of Addictive Disease, 21*(1), 45–60.

Walton-Moss, B., Campbell, J. C., & Sharps, P. W. (in press). Ethnic group specific risk factors for intimate partner femicide. *Homicide Studies.*

Websdale, N. (1999). *Understanding domestic homicide.* Boston: Northeastern University Press.

Weisz, A. N., Tolman, R. M., & Saunders, D. G. (2000). Assessing the risk of severe domestic violence: The importance of survivors' predictions. *Journal of Interpersonal Violence, 15,* 75–90.

Zawitz, M. W. (1994). *Violence between intimates.* Washington, DC: Bureau of Justice Statistics.

CHAPTER 2

Prediction Issues for Practitioners

Joel S. Milner and Jacquelyn C. Campbell

Practitioners often are called upon to predict the dangerousness of clients. Because the situations in which predictions are made vary greatly, some authors have suggested that distinctions be made between formal and informal predictions (e.g., Werner, Rose, & Yesavage, 1990). *Formal prediction* refers to views expressed by professionals in hearings and court proceedings that influence sentencing, parole, and custody decisions. *Informal prediction* refers to comments made by practitioners in clinical situations with criminal justice system officials, health care professionals, victim advocates, and potential victims. Regardless of whether the prediction is formal or informal, practitioners are obligated to be as accurate as possible and to have considered the ethical dilemmas of (a) confidentiality versus warning and (b) protection of individual rights versus the collective good.

Although many practitioners may be reluctant to make predictions because of problems with prediction accuracy and ethical considerations, they are constantly under pressure to do so by formal systems, other professionals, clients, and clients' families. For example, with increasing frequency practitioners are being asked to serve as expert witnesses in cases of sexual and spousal abuse. Although practitioners may be able to avoid becoming involved in formal predictions, there still are legal and ethical mandates for practitioners to make informal predictions of dangerousness, such as when they inform potential victims. Thus practitioners involved in work with violent or potentially violent clients have a great need for understanding the nature, process, and research status of prediction.

CLINICAL VERSUS STATISTICAL PREDICTION STRATEGIES

When discussing different types of prediction, it is useful to make a distinction between clinical and statistical prediction. Miller and Morris (1988) describe *clinical prediction* as being based on professional training, professional experience, and observation of a particular client. Clinical predictions are subjective or intuitive in nature, and may or may not be organized into a structured format. *Statistical prediction* involves predicting an individual's behavior on the basis of how others have acted in similar situations (actuarial) or on an individual's similarity to members of violent groups. Such prediction is based on statistical models (e.g., additive linear models, clustering models, contingency table analysis) derived from research and includes the use of risk factor instruments (e.g., Gottfredson & Gottfredson, 1988; Miller & Morris, 1988; Ruscio, 1998).

Clinical predictions have been criticized for producing decisions that are inconsistent, inequitable, biased, and inaccurate (e.g., Milner, Murphy, Valle, & Tolliver, 1998; Odeh, Zeiss, & Huss, 2006). Further, clinical predictions may lack accountability because the criteria and rationale used in the assessment process are not explicit. Although there still are debates (e.g., Baumann, Law, Sheets, Reid, & Graham, 2006; Johnson, 2006), the consensus of opinion is that statistical prediction is more accurate than clinical prediction. Thus, whenever possible, we strongly recommend using statistical procedures to increase the accuracy of clinical prediction.

A summary of the criteria commonly used in the different types of prediction of violent behavior is presented in Table 2.1. As indicated, informal clinical prediction often occurs without the assistance of validated instruments by using the kinds of models outlined in Chapter 1. In formal prediction, however, statistical methods and/or risk instruments that meet certain psychometric standards should be used. To this end, more than a decade ago Monahan (1993) emphasized the need for "familiarity with basic concepts in risk assessment (e.g., predictor and criterion variables, true and false positives and negatives, decision rules, base rates)" (p. 247). In this chapter we concentrate on issues related to the use of instruments for prediction. Other statistical prediction methods have been discussed elsewhere (for overviews, see Gottfredson & Gottfredson, 1988; Ruscio, 1998).

TABLE 2.1   Approaches Commonly Used in the Formal and Informal Prediction of Violent Behavior

	Formal	Informal
Clinical	1 & 2	1
Statistical	3	2

1. Clinical judgment through interview and other subjective assessments.
2. Risk factor identification is used. Construct and validity data are needed to support the use of a risk factor instrument.
3. Dichotomous/Criterion/Cutoff scores are used. The assessment instrument provides a score designated as the criterion or cutoff that is used to place an individual into one category or another. Concurrent and future predictive validity data and individual classification rates are needed.

Note: Although this table is a summary of procedures used in the clinical and statistical prediction of violence, in all cases multiple data sources should be used in making predictions regarding violence. Further, when formal statistical prediction is possible, a single test score must never be used to make a prediction.

LEGAL ISSUES AND PREDICTION

Practitioners involved in violence prediction must be aware of both the limitations in their ability to predict violence and the evolving legal duties to warn and protect others from the violent acts of their clients. Following the landmark *Tarasoff v. Regents of the University of California* (1976) decision, which defined a broader professional responsibility for informing and protecting individuals from possible client violence, there was a dramatic expansion by the courts of professionals' responsibility to inform and protect third parties. In contrast, in the decade of the 1990s, there was "a substantial retreat from the original Tarasoff principle" (Felthous & Kachigian, 2001). A review of the Tarasoff principle and subsequent expansion and more recent restrictions and rejections of the Tarasoff principle are available elsewhere (e.g., Behnke, Perlin, & Bernstein, 2005; Walcott, Cerundolo, & Beck, 2001; see also Chapter 1). In addition, practitioners must be mindful of related rulings on patient-client confidentiality that include social workers engaged in psychotherapy (e.g., *Jaffee v. Redmond;* see Colledge, Zeigler, Hemmens, & Hodge, 2000; Mitrevski & Chamberlain, 2006). Although a description of recent changes regarding legal obligations to warn and protect is beyond the scope of this chapter, practitioners working with violent clients must continually inform themselves about legislative and judicial changes in their obligation to warn and protect third parties from a potentially violent client.

ETHICAL ISSUES AND PREDICTION

In addition to the legal duty to warn, professional organizations of psychiatrists and psychologists have standards of practice that state the therapist must warn potential victims. For example, the American Medical Association's Principles of Medical Ethics mandates that physicians protect potential victims of patients by taking action, such as notifying law enforcement agencies. Even without organizationally prescribed professional standards, clinicians have ethical responsibilities to persons in physical danger (see Gutheil, 2001, for a discussion of ethical considerations related to when a warning may be ethically justified).

Prediction also involves the possibility (a) that one's own biases will influence one's judgment and (b) of subjecting a person to unfair criminal justice penalties on the basis of an inaccurate prediction. As a result of these dilemmas, clinicians often desire fail-safe prediction instruments so that no judgment is necessary. The reality, of course, is that statistical methods are in various stages of development and that their ability to correctly screen violent and nonviolent individuals will never be totally accurate. Thus the practitioner's knowledge of clinical assessment remains an extremely important adjunct to any statistical prediction. Instrumentation can be a valuable source of objective data, provided that prior use and testing of a measure have supported its reliability and validity.

The legal and ethical responsibility of clinicians includes becoming as knowledgeable as possible about the dynamics of violence, particularly in terms of potential for further dangerousness. In addition, clinicians need to know about instruments that measure dangerousness in specific areas (e.g., child abuse and spousal abuse, as opposed to general aggressiveness or pathology) and the limits of their use, topics covered in Chapters 3 through 6. In the remainder of this chapter we discuss how one evaluates the psychometric properties of risk assessment instruments.

PSYCHOMETRIC ISSUES IN CLINICAL PRACTICE

The belief that professionals dealing with violent clients need to increase their knowledge of measurement issues is supported by research findings. For example, Milner (1989) surveyed 550 administrators, researchers, and practitioners in the family violence field to determine their knowledge of appropriate uses of the Child Abuse Potential (CAP) Inventory, a screening scale for child physical abuse (Milner, 1986, 1994, 2004). The survey revealed that a substantial number of professionals suggested applications for the CAP Inventory that were inappropriate or not supported by validity data. Milner concluded that an increase in professional knowledge of the proper use of child abuse screening instruments should accompany the development of such instruments or the use of family violence screening instruments should be restricted to those who have credentials (e.g., licensed psychologists) to help ensure an adequate knowledge of measurement issues.

In an attempt to increase the practitioner's knowledge of psychometric issues, we discuss some of the traditional psychometric requirements for tests and measures. The reader should note that a comprehensive set of standards has been developed to guide the practitioner in the evaluation and use of test instruments. Psychometric and practice standards are provided in the publication *Standards for Educational and Psychological Testing* (American Psychological Association, 1999). This document includes sections that describe the responsibilities of the test constructor, the test publisher, and the test user.

As standards have evolved, the trend has been toward increasing the responsibility of the test user for the determination that a test is appropriate for a given application. Further, when the test constructor or test publisher does not provide data that support a specific test application (e.g., violence prediction) and the test user nevertheless makes the application, the test user is responsible for providing research evidence to support the new application. Documentation also is needed when the test application is not new but the population under investigation has not been previously studied. In this case, prior to test use, the test user is responsible for collecting data to indicate that the test is still appropriate when used with the new participant population.

APPROACHES TO DEVELOPING PREDICTIVE INSTRUMENTS

Ideally the development of an instrument or test is based on a well-defined, empirically validated model that describes etiologic variables. Constructs from the model are used to define the content domains, or areas to be covered by the proposed instrument. Guided by the content domains, a large pool of items is developed and administered to criterion and matched comparison groups. The criterion group is chosen to exemplify or "have" the characteristic being measured. Then an item analysis is conducted to determine the best predictors. After item cross-validation, which involves replicating the predictive ability of the items by using another sample of criterion and comparison participants, factor analysis can be conducted to provide descriptive factors. Then it is determined whether the total score or some configuration of factor scores most effectively discriminates the criterion participants from comparison participants.

In cases in which explanatory theories are lacking, a combination of rational and empirical approaches can be used to develop test items (e.g., Edwards, 1970). In this approach, different theoretical perspectives and empirical studies are used to develop an array of content domains to guide test construction. This technique often is called a "shotgun" approach to test development, wherein all possibly relevant domains are used to guide item development. When there are no well-developed models, however, this technique provides a method for test construction that can result in the successful development of a risk instrument. A drawback of developing a measure without a guiding explanatory model is that important etiologic variables may be omitted from the content domains used to develop the assessment items.

Fortunately, for a screening instrument to be successful, not all content domains have to be used in the development of the test. Indeed, from a psychometric perspective, the predictive factors need not be related directly to the etiology. A subset of the descriptive factors, whether causal or marker variables, often can be found that are reliably correlated with the criterion behavior (e.g., physical abuse) and that can predict the behavior. Although this approach frequently is criticized, in reality most measures are constructed by using only a subset of the content domains related to the predicted behavior.

TEST RELIABILITY

Although many types of reliability are mentioned in the psychometric literature, instrument reliability is of two major types: *internal consistency* and *temporal stability*. Internal consistency and temporal stability reliabilities are statistically represented by correlation coefficients.

Internal Consistency

Estimates of *internal consistency,* or *item consistency,* provide information on the equivalence, or homogeneity, of the test items. This equivalence provides an estimate of the degree to which the test items are all measuring the same construct. Internal consistency estimates usually are presented as alpha coefficients. High internal consistency indicates that a test is measuring a specific construct, such as depression. Low internal consistency suggests that more than one construct or a multidimensional construct, such as self-concept, is being assessed.

Internal consistency estimates are affected by test length. A scale with few test items (e.g., five items) must be very homogeneous to have high (e.g., .90) internal consistency, whereas a scale with a large number of test items (e.g., 100) actually may include a variety of different but related items (e.g., distress, anxiety, impulsiveness) and still have a relatively high internal consistency. Test reliability is important because it sets the upper limits for test validity; that is, on average, test validity of an instrument cannot be higher than the internal consistency of the test. In most cases test validity estimates will be lower, sometimes markedly lower, than the internal consistency estimates.

Temporal Stability

The *temporal stability* of a test score indicates the degree of test score stability, or how similar test scores are over a specified time period. High levels of temporal stability suggest that the construct being measured tends to be stable over time and that the test is measuring the same construct in the same way across time. Temporal stability estimates are calculated by correlating test scores obtained from the same participant at two points in time. Thus temporal stability estimates are represented by test-retest correlations for different time intervals, such as 1-week, 1-month, and 1-year test-retest intervals.

The expected degree of temporal stability of a test score should be high if the test purports to measure a personality trait because these personality characteristics are expected to be stable across time. In contrast the level of acceptable temporal stability of a test score may be relatively modest or low if the test is designed to measure a personality state that is expected to change across time. So the level of test-retest reliability, or temporal stability, should vary as a function of the conceptualization of the construct (trait or state) under investigation.

When evaluating the temporal stability of a test, the extent of gain scores is important to note. Gain scores describe test score increases that occur at the second testing, relative to the first testing. Most psychological tests tend to have slightly higher scores at the second testing. Thus, when test-retest reliabilities are presented, the test score means and standard deviations obtained at each test period should be published so that the practitioner can evaluate the size of any gain score.

Test-retest reliabilities and gain scores are of particular concern in certain test applications. For example, in research designs in which multiple evaluations are made at different time intervals, knowledge of the test's temporal stability is critical. Examples of such studies include pretreatment and posttreatment evaluation research and longitudinal victim effects studies, in which the same measures are administered repeatedly, usually at fixed time intervals. In these designs, only tests with appropriate temporal stability and modest gain scores for the time periods should be used.

TEST VALIDITY

Validity data provide information on the extent to which a test is adequate for the intended use. In the validation process the inferences made from test scores, not the actual test scores, are validated. As part of the investigation of the psychometric qualities of a test, different types of validity data should be accumulated. It is the accumulated validity evidence from many studies conducted by different investigators, not the evidence from any single study, that allows the user to determine whether the instrument measures what it purports to measure. Ideally, specific validity data for a particular type of application are accumulated so that the mass of evidence supports or does not support a given test application.

Frequently test validity data may indicate that a test is appropriate for one use with a given population, while data may not be sufficient to support the same application with another population or for another application with the same population. For example, a prediction instrument may have data from several sources that support predicting future sexual child abuse in White, male perpetrator samples but have little or no data supporting the use of the instrument to predict recidivism in African American groups.

Further, no test should ever be said to be "valid" for its intended use. Test validation is a matter of degree of validity for certain applications with specific populations. Validation is an ongoing process and never a completed task. Test reviews or advertisements that indicate a test is "valid" or has been "fully validated" are inappropriate and misleading. More appropriate is the review or advertisement that indicates substantial data exist demonstrating the test has some degree of validity for a specific application with a specific population or populations. Further, the supporting psychometric data for a test should be available to the test user and other interested professionals in the published literature and in a technical manual. If the relevant validity information is not readily available, the author of the instrument should be contacted to determine whether such information exists.

Although different types of test validity have been described, three broad categories of test validity, which contain some overlap, usually are of interest. These are *content, construct,* and *predictive* (post hoc, concurrent, future type) *validity*. Each of these categories is discussed in the following sections.

Content Validity

The *content validity* of a test refers to the extent to which the test items represent a specific content domain. As previously discussed, the content domain typically is defined by the theoretical model on which the test is based. In cases in which no model is used to guide the development of test items, some rational or empirical approach is used to guide the item development, and this approach serves to define the content domains. In either case, the approach used defines the domain or domains that must be sampled adequately during test construction.

The extent to which the test items represent the guiding conceptual domains indicates the degree of content validity. Thus the procedures that guided the construction of the test items and the face validity of the items are used to inform the user about the degree of content validity. Content validity can be demonstrated by obtaining evaluations of items from experts in the field. In addition, content validity is supported if the test scores are correlated with other measures of constructs representing the content domains used to develop the test items.

Construct Validity

Overlapping somewhat with content validity, *construct validity* refers to the extent to which the underlying constructs assumed to be measured by the test actually are measured. Construct data provide verification of what initially was theoretically or intuitively assumed during the test item construction. Construct validity is supported by the accumulation of data that verify that the characteristics the instrument was designed to measure are indeed measured. In addition, development of a large array of different types of construct validity data provides a mosaic of information that allows the test user to understand what the instrument is measuring. Such information serves to assist the user in making more appropriate test score interpretations.

In general, two broad types of construct validity exist: *convergent validity* and *discriminant validity*. Convergent validity data are generated when factors thought to be related to the test scores are shown to be related. Discriminant validity data are generated when factors believed to be extraneous to the test scores are found to be unrelated. Convergent and discriminant validity can be demonstrated by a variety of techniques, such as comparison of test scores with other test scores, with relationships demonstrated only where relationships are expected; demonstration of expected relationships between test scores and different criterion and comparison groups; conceptually congruent factor analysis; and test data from program evaluations that show the test scores are sensitive to treatment effects.

Predictive Validity

Test *predictive validity,* or *criterion validity,* consists of three types: post hoc, concurrent, and future type (e.g., Nunnally, 1978). *Post hoc prediction* refers to the prediction of a condition in the past. *Concurrent prediction* refers to the prediction of a condition that presently exists. *Future prediction* refers to the prediction of a condition or event that has not yet occurred, which includes both a first occurrence and recidivism. Future prediction, therefore, involves "forecasting" the occurrence of future events on the basis of present test scores. Each of these three types of prediction is needed in the detection and prevention of violence.

Post hoc prediction is very difficult, and this type of validity data is rarely available for a test. The major problem in post hoc prediction is that the test data are collected after the occurrence of the behavior. Although a temporal separation between testing and the predicted behavior also exists for future prediction (as discussed later), more problems exist for post hoc prediction. Not only can random intervening variables affect test scores and reduce the predictive relationship, but when violence does occur, consequences often result from the occurrence of the behavior. In some cases legal intervention will occur or treatment will be provided. In the case of family violence, children may be removed or a wife may leave. These and other direct consequences of the violence can affect the personality and interactional characteristics of the perpetrator. Therefore subsequent testing of the violent perpetrator may not represent the conditions present at the time of the abuse, making post hoc prediction difficult.

Concurrent predictive validity is especially important when a test is used to place an individual in a particular group (e.g., currently abusive). Although concurrent predictive validity data are more often available for a test, most of these data are expressed in terms of group differences, as opposed to individual classification rates. That is, test data typically only indicate that a test shows significant group differences between a criterion group (e.g., child physical abusers) and a comparison group (e.g., nonabusers).

Although group differences must exist if a test is capable of individual discrimination, the finding that a test shows significant group differences between criterion and comparison groups does not alone mean that the test has acceptable individual classification ability. Further, many studies that compare groups do not match the criterion and comparison groups on demographic variables, a shortcoming that increases the likelihood that group differences will be found but for the wrong reasons. In test validation studies where criterion and comparison groups are not matched and group differences are found, it is not known whether the group differences are due to the criterion variable or to group demographic differences or to both factors.

What are needed to demonstrate adequate individual predictive validity are the individual classification rates for test scores based on well-defined criteria and demographically matched comparison groups. Although some risk assessment procedures use demographic characteristics as risk markers (such as single parent status, age, education level), this profiling approach results in numerous ethical problems and assures the overinclusion of those with the characteristics in the risk group (even though they are not at risk) and the underinclusion of those who are at risk but do not have the selected demographic characteristics.

A remaining problem is that reported individual classification rates often are based on a statistical procedure known as *discriminant analysis*. Although discriminant analysis is appropriate for providing initial estimates of individual predictive validity, this procedure provides optimal classification rates for each sample tested because it reweights the item scores in each new analysis. Therefore, as individual classification data accumulate, some of the data should be obtained by using the test instrument standard scoring procedure designed for field use. Some decrease in the individual correct classification rates can be expected when a standard scoring procedure is used across a variety of demographically different populations.

When individual classification rates are available, the test user should note carefully the percentage of false positive classifications (nonabusers labeled as abusive) and false negative classifications (abusers labeled as nonabusive). Related to these estimates are the sensitivity and specificity of the test. Test sensitivity is the percentage of correct classifications of abusers; test specificity is the percentage of correct classifications of nonabusers. These four outcomes expressed in terms of risk assessment for violence are presented in Table 2.2.

In most cases in which predictive validity is provided, it is the concurrent type. Future predictive validity, often the most desirable type of validity when violence is under study, is rarely provided. In the few cases in which these data are available, the validity data are typically modest or not significant. In fairness to test developers, it should be mentioned that future prediction is very problematic not only because of the difficulties involved in the design of a predictive instrument but also because numerous variables can intervene between the testing session and the predicted event. These intervening variables may increase or decrease the likelihood of the event, thus reducing the test's predictive ability.

TABLE 2.2   Types of Individual Classification Outcomes

	Actual risk status	
Screened Risk	Client at risk	Client not at risk
Client at risk	A	B
Client not at risk	C	D

A. Correct classification of at-risk status (sensitivity)
B. Misclassification of risk status (false positive classification)
C. Misclassification of nonrisk status (false negative classification)
D. Correct classification of nonrisk status (specificity)

OTHER MEASUREMENT ISSUES

In addition to the determination that adequate reliability and validity data exist to support a desired test application, a number of other measurement issues must be considered when a test is used to assess interpersonal violence. Several of the more important measurement considerations are (a) the possibility of participant response distortion, (b) the availability of appropriate test norms, (c) the size of the standard error of measurement, and (d) the estimated violence base rates.

Response Distortions

A major issue related to the use of self-report approaches, including both interview and questionnaire assessment, is the possibility that individuals will distort their responses to questions. Response distortions include faking-good, faking-bad, and random response behavior. Faking-good behavior is related to the respondent's attempt to distort responses in a socially desirable manner or to present himself or herself in a favorable light. Faking-bad behavior is related to the respondent's attempt to distort responses in a socially undesirable manner and to present himself or herself in an unfavorable light. Random response behavior is related to the respondent giving responses that do not represent responses to the item content. Random responding may be due to a variety of factors, such as a deliberate desire to avoid revealing personal data or an inability to understand item content. A more complete discussion of possible causes of the three types of response distortions is available elsewhere (e.g., Milner, 2006).

Because response distortions can render test data meaningless, professionals need to include in their assessment package some measures of response distortions (e.g., faking-good, faking-bad, random response indexes from existing tests such as the Child Abuse Potential [CAP] Inventory [Milner, 1986]). This inclusion is especially important in the assessment of violence perpetrators because these respondents often are motivated to distort responses made to professionals investigating violence.

Test Norms

The interpretation of a test score is aided by the availability of test norms. Norm scores (e.g., test score means, standard deviations) should be available for well-defined populations. The test manual should indicate the year in which the norm data were collected and provide detailed descriptions of the methods used to collect the norm data and the demographic characteristics of the norm group.

Norms may represent local or regional populations or a national probability sampling. In addition, norm data should be presented as a function of gender, ethnic background, age, marital status, educational level, socioeconomic level, number of children, and so on. Thus the test user should expect the test manual to provide numerous test norms so that he or she can inspect the norm data for possible moderator (demographic) variable effects. For example, on the Family Environment Scale (FES) (Moos & Moos, 1986) the norm scores for the family conflict scale vary by more than 100% on the basis of family size (e.g., two family members, conflict score $M = 2.11$; five family members, conflict score $M = 4.78$). In this case, failure to consider the number of family members could result in a dramatic misunderstanding of the meaning of the FES conflict score. The problem is actually more serious on this and other tests because often several moderating variables must be considered.

Although national norms are not available for most tests, norms representing the population from which the respondent was drawn usually are required in order to give meaning to the obtained test score. The norm test scores provide population-based values that enable the user to interpret the obtained test scores in relation to those obtained from a similar participant group. Finally, the types of norm values needed can vary as a function of the test application. Thus the practitioner must determine which norm data are needed for the proper interpretation of the test score and whether these norms are available, rather than simply use whatever norms are presented in the test manual.

Standard Error of Measurement

The test user must be aware that all test scores contain measurement error. An estimate of measurement error, the *standard error of measurement* (SEM), should be available for each test scale. The SEM provides an estimate of the variation of the obtained score from the true score. Because the SEM is a standard deviation, it can be used to set a confidence interval around the obtained score so that the range of scores that includes the true score can be known. The SEM is especially important in the prediction of interpersonal violence when test cutoff scores are used to classify the examinee and the examinee's obtained test score is near the test cutoff score. The examinee's obtained test score should be sufficiently beyond the test cutoff score, as determined by the SEM, so that the interpretation that the test score is elevated is less likely to be the result of chance.

Violence Base Rates

Professionals need to be aware of the role of base rates in the prediction of behavior. In the prediction of child abuse or any other violent behavior, the base rate affects the amount of incremental prediction added by a measure in the detection of the behavior under investigation. Optimal increases in prediction occur when the base rates are 50%, which means that 50% of the sample or population are the criterion cases (perpetrators of violence). For example, if a test has an 80% correct classification rate for both abusive and nonabusive parents and the test is used in a situation in which 50% of the participants tested are abusive (base rate of 50%), then the classification rate is 80% for each group. If the test is administered to 100 participants, then 40 abusers (80% of 50 abusers) and 40 nonabusers (80% of nonabusers) will be classified correctly, resulting in an 80% overall classification rate and an equal number of false positive and false negative classifications.

When the base rates are lower than 50%, the usefulness of the test in the selection of who is abusive decreases to the point where the test may be inappropriate. For example, if the same test with an 80% correct classification rate is used in a situation in which only 5% of the participants tested are abusive (base rate of 5%) in a group of 100 participants, then the ratio of false positive and false negative classifications will vary dramatically. In light of the 80% correct classification rate for abusers, 4 of the 5 abusers will be classified correctly; however, only 80% of the 95 nonabusers will be classified correctly, resulting in 19 false positive classifications. Thus, overall, 23 participants (4 correct abuser classifications and 19 false positive classifications) will be indicated as abusive, with only 4 of the 23 actually being abusive. This result means that only 17.4% of those classified as abusers are actually abusive, with 82.6% of those labeled abusive being false positive classifications.

It also is true, however, that the number of correct classifications in the 77 participants classified as nonabusers will increase. In this example only 1 of the 77 participants classified as nonabusers will be a false positive classification, resulting in a 98.7% correct classification rate for those labeled nonabusers. Thus, as the base rate decreases, the percentage of false positive and false negative classifications will change dramatically from the classification rates derived from studies in which 50% of the participants are abusive and non-abusive. It is always important, therefore, for the professional to estimate the base rate for the population under study and to determine the relative utility of the test for the intended application.

SUMMARY

As increasing numbers of measures are developed for use in assessing violence potential, professionals will be required to discriminate between those tests that have some utility and those that should be avoided. As previously noted, the responsibility for making adequate test selection and application is increasingly the responsibility of the test user. This responsibility requires that practitioners increase and maintain their knowledge of psychometric issues related to test selection and use.

Clinicians can avoid making formal predictions in the courtroom, but clients who are perpetrators and victims of child, spouse, and sexual abuse are almost impossible to avoid, given the rates of violent behavior in our society. Thus clinicians must be able to make reasonably accurate assessments of the potential for future dangerousness in order to fulfill their ethical and legal mandates to warn and protect potential victims. Clinical expertise (appropriate academic, clinical, and legal training, knowledge of the risk literature), coupled with some form of statistical prediction, allows the greatest accuracy of prediction at the present time.

EVALUATING AN INSTRUMENT

As an example of evaluating the utility of an instrument for prediction, we examine the psychometric properties of the Index of Spouse Abuse (ISA) (Hudson & McIntosh, 1981). Although not specifically designed as a prediction instrument, the ISA might be considered a potentially useful instrument for predicting the seriousness of wife abuse. The ISA is a self-report scale designed to be completed by the female victim of spousal abuse. It assesses verbal, emotional, sexual, and physical aggression and was designed to evaluate treatment progress in identified spousal abuse victims. The ISA provides two subscale scores: a severity of physical abuse score (ISA-P) and a severity of nonphysical abuse score (ISA-NP).

Hudson and McIntosh (1981) reported internal consistency reliability estimates (alphas) of .90 and .91 for the ISA-P subscale and .94 to .97 for the ISA-NP subscale. In a sample of African American, Latino, and White pregnant women, McFarlane, Parker, Soeken, and Bullock (1992) reported internal consistency estimates of .87 for the ISA-P subscale and .93 for ISA-NP subscale. Similarly Campbell, Campbell, King, Parker, and Ryan (2001) found adequate internal consistency reliabilities for an African American sample. These data support the view that each of the ISA subscales is unidimensional. No information is available on the temporal stability (test-retest reliability) of the ISA scales.

The construct validity of the ISA subscales is supported by a factor analysis that yielded the two expected factors (Hudson & McIntosh, 1981). Hudson and McIntosh also reported a number of correlations that indicate the ISA subscales are not associated with factors thought to have relatively little relationship with spousal abuse (discriminant validity) and are associated with factors thought to be related to spousal abuse (convergent validity), albeit some of the expected correlations were modest. In another study, Campbell (see Chapter 5, this volume) reported a correlation of .767 between the ISA-P and the Danger Assessment scale (DA). The DA was designed to assess the risk of homicide in battering relationships. This finding provides support for the view that higher ISA-P scores are associated with more serious wife abuse. The DA is a recently developed instrument, however, and it is unclear to what extent elevated scores on the DA are associated with homicide, which is a low base rate event and therefore is very difficult to predict.

Hudson and McIntosh (1981) reported on the classification ability of the ISA. They reported classification errors for both of the ISA subscales to be 9.3% for a group of abused and nonabused participants. These rates were found when optimal cutting scores were determined after examination of the cumulative frequency distributions for the scores obtained from the abused and nonabused participants. Although these results are encouraging, they need to be cross-validated. It is not known to what extent the same cutting scores would discriminate in a different sample. Further, in the description of the nonabused participants it was not clear how it was determined that the nonabused women were "free from any clinically significant partner or spouse abuse" (Hudson & McIntosh, 1981, p. 876). In another study, McFarlane et al. (1992) also found that the ISA could discriminate abused from nonabused pregnant women, where abuse was identified by a short structured interview. However, in this study there is the possibility of tautological effects resulting from asking the same or similar questions twice.

Little additional information is available on the ISA because it has not been widely used in published studies of wife abuse. Further, a new version of the scale has been published. The new scale, which has been renamed the Partner

Abuse Scales, also contains two subscales (marketed as two separate instruments) for physical and nonphysical abuse. Although the authors indicate that the new scales have high reliability and good content and factor validity, along with other supportive construct validity, not all of the research supporting these claims has been published (Hudson, 1990). Support for reliability and construct validity of the PAS has been reported by Attala (1994) and colleagues (Attala, Hudson, & McSweeney, 1994), but they found that a lower cutoff score indicated abuse than that suggested by Hudson (1990).

In summary, the original ISA scales appear to have adequate internal consistency. However, no data are available on the temporal stability (test-retest reliability) of the ISA scales. This is an important omission. If test items represent constructs that are not stable across time, this variation will make the prediction of future events difficult, if not impossible. Although the ISA was not designed with future prediction in mind, it still is important to know the temporal stability of the ISA across different time intervals because the ISA scale was designed for use in treatment evaluation. If the ISA scores are highly variable across time, it will be difficult to show that score changes across the treatment period are due to treatment effects, and not to test instability. Noteworthy is the fact that initial discriminant validity data are available for concurrent prediction of abuse and nonabuse group membership. Further, cut scores have been established for classification purposes, but there is some disagreement in the literature about the validity of the cut scores of the revised ISA, the PAS (Attala, 1994). Therefore, the cut scores need to be cross-validated on additional samples. Finally, additional criterion data (especially behavioral data) are needed to support the view that higher scores on the ISA scales are predictive of more severe levels of spousal abuse. This support requires some evidence that the ISA scales have interval scale characteristics.

REFERENCES

American Psychological Association. (1999). *Standards for educational and psychological testing*. Washington, DC: Author.

Attala, J. M. (1994). Risk identification of abused women participating in a Women, Infants, and Children program. *Health Care for Women International, 15*, 587–597.

Attala, J. M., Hudson, W. W., & McSweeney, M. (1994). A partial validation of two short-form Partner Abuse Scales. *Women & Health, 2*, 125–139.

Baumann, D. J., Law, R. J., Sheets, J., Reid, G., & Graham, C. J. (2006). Remarks concerning the importance of evaluation actuarial risk assessment models: A rejoinder to Will Johnson. *Children and Youth Services Review, 28*, 715–725.

Behnke, S. H., Perlin, M. L., & Bernstein, M. D. (2005). Tarasoff and the duty to protect. *NYS Psychologist, 17*, 21–26.

Campbell, D., Campbell, J., King, C., Parker, B., & Ryan, J. (2001). The reliability and factor structure of the Index of Spouse Abuse with African-American women. In K. D. O'Leary & R. D. Maiuro (Eds.), *Psychological abuse in violent domestic relations* (pp. 101–118). New York: Springer Publishing.

Colledge, D., Zeigler, F., Hemmens, C., & Hodge, C. (2000). What's up doc? *Jaffee v. Redmond* and the psychotherapeutic privilege in criminal justice. *Journal of Criminal Justice, 28,* 1–11.

Edwards, A. L. (1970). *The measurement of personality traits by scales and inventories.* New York: Holt, Rinehart & Winston.

Felthous, A. R., & Kachigian, C. (2001). To warn and to control: Two distinct legal obligations or variations on a single duty to protect? *Behavioral Sciences & the Law, 19,* 355–373.

Gottfredson, D. M., & Gottfredson, S. D. (1988). Stakes and risks in the prediction of violent criminal behavior. *Violence and Victims, 3,* 247–262.

Gutheil, T. G. (2001). Moral justification for Tarasoff-type warnings and breach of confidentiality: A clinician's perspective. *Behavioral Sciences & the Law, 19,* 345–353.

Hudson, W. W. (1990). *Partner Abuse Scales.* Tempe, AZ: Walmyr.

Hudson, W. W., & McIntosh, S. R. (1981). The assessment of spouse abuse: Two quantifiable dimensions. *Journal of Marriage and the Family, 43,* 873–885.

Johnson, W. (2006). The risk assessment wars: A commentary response to "Evaluating the effectiveness of actuarial risk assessment models" by Donald Baumann, J. Randolph Law, Janess Sheets, Grant Reid, and J. Christopher Graham. *Children and Youth Services Review, 27,* pp. 465–490. *Children and Youth Services Review, 28,* 701–714.

McFarlane, J., Parker, B., Soeken, K., & Bullock, L. (1992). Assessing for abuse during pregnancy: Frequency and extent of injuries and associated entry into prenatal care. *Journal of the American Medical Association, 267,* 3176–3198.

Miller, M., & Morris, N. (1988). Predictions of dangerousness: An argument for limited use. *Violence and Victims, 3,* 263–284.

Milner, J. S. (1986). *The Child Abuse Potential Inventory: Manual* (2nd ed.). Webster, NC: Psytec.

Milner, J. S. (1989). Applications of the Child Abuse Potential Inventory. *Journal of Clinical Psychology, 45,* 450–454.

Milner, J. S. (1994). Assessing physical child abuse risk: The Child Abuse Potential Inventory. *Clinical Psychology Review, 14,* 547–583.

Milner, J. S. (2004). The Child Abuse Potential (CAP) Inventory. In M. L. Hilsenroth & D. L. Segal (Eds.), *Comprehensive handbook of psychological assessment: Vol. 2. Personality assessment* (pp. 237–246). Hoboken, NJ: John Wiley & Sons.

Milner, J. S. (2006). *An interpretive manual for the Child Abuse Potential Inventory.* DeKalb, IL: Psytec.

Milner, J. S., Murphy, W. D., Valle, L. A., & Tolliver, R. M. (1998). Assessment issues in child abuse evaluations. In J. R. Lutzker (Ed.), *Handbook of child abuse research and treatment* (pp. 75–115). New York: Plenum Press.

Mitrevski, J. P., & Chamberlain, J. R. (2006). Psychotherapist-patient privilege: Applying *Jaffee v. Redmond*: Communications to a psychotherapist are not privileged if they occur outside the course of diagnosis or treatment. *Journal of the American Academy of Psychiatry and the Law, 34,* 245–246.

Monahan, J. (1993). Limiting therapist exposure to Tarasoff liability: Guidelines for risk containment. *American Psychologist, 48,* 242–250.

Moos, R. H., & Moos, B. S. (1986). *Family Environment Scale Manual* (2nd ed.). Palo Alto, CA: Consulting Psychologists Press.

Nunnally, J. C. (1978). *Psychometric theory.* New York: McGraw-Hill.

Odeh, M. S., Zeiss, R. A., & Huss, M. T. (2006). Cues they use: Clinicians' endorsement of risk cues in predictions of dangerousness. *Behavioral Sciences & the Law, 24,* 147–156.

Ruscio, J. (1998). Information integration in child welfare cases: An introduction to statistical decision making. *Child Maltreatment, 3,* 143–156.

Tarasoff v. Regents of the University of California. 551 P.2d 334 (1976), vacating 529 P.2d 553 (1974).

Walcott, D. M., Cerundolo, P., & Beck, J. C. (2001). Current analysis of the Tarasoff duty: An evolution towards the limitation of the duty to protect. *Behavioral Sciences & the Law, 19,* 325–343

Werner, P. D., Rose, T. L., & Yesavage, J. A. (1990). Aspects of consensus in clinical prediction of imminent violence. *Journal of Clinical Psychology, 46,* 534–538.

CHAPTER 3

Child Physical Abuse Assessment: Perpetrator Evaluation

Joel S. Milner

Each year, approximately three million child maltreatment referrals are made to social services agencies in the United States (U.S. Department of Health and Human Services, 2006). Collectively, these referrals involve more than five and one-half million children. In 2004, the most recent year in which official data are available, 63% of all referrals were accepted for investigation and, among these, approximately 30% were confirmed for child maltreatment (U.S. Department of Health and Human Services, 2006).[1] Although the majority of all investigated referrals were confirmed for child neglect, about 17.5% were confirmed for child physical abuse, the focus of the present chapter.

When child maltreatment referrals are accepted for investigation by state departments of social services, child protective services workers are required to collect assessment data and to render a timely decision regarding the occurrence of child maltreatment. During this assessment process, protective services workers attempt to substantiate the report and, if substantiated, to identify the perpetrator. Unfortunately, in many child maltreatment investigations, time and resource limitations require that protective services workers make decisions based on a limited amount of assessment data.

45

If child maltreatment is confirmed, case workers must estimate the likelihood of future maltreatment when they decide to leave the child in or remove the child from the home. In situations where the child is removed, case workers often must determine if and when the child should be returned. Although more case data are usually available at the time this decision is made, the assessment task remains difficult because, when they are making a decision about returning a child, case workers must estimate (predict) the likelihood of future events (e.g., re-abuse).

Recidivism (e.g., likelihood of re-abuse) assessments are especially difficult because intervening variables (factors that occur after the assessment) can affect future parenting behavior. Thus, after detection and intervention, assessment data may indicate a low risk of recidivism. However, later events (e.g., new stressors) may increase the risk potential even though the low-risk determination after intervention was a valid estimate at the time of the evaluation. While not always possible, one obvious method of reducing recidivism prediction errors caused by intervening events is to conduct additional risk assessments at future dates.

RISK ASSESSMENT IN PRIMARY, SECONDARY, AND TERTIARY INTERVENTION

Although the above discussion of caretaker assessment has focused on the risk assessment activities of protective service providers, the utility and purpose of risk assessment varies as a function of the type of intervention. Traditionally, prevention/intervention programs have been divided into three general types: primary, secondary, and tertiary prevention.

Primary prevention efforts usually assume that all parents are at risk for child abuse, so assessment procedures for determining risk status are not necessary. Primary prevention programs, which attempt to prevent child abuse prior to its occurrence, often focus on treating beliefs, practices, and conditions in the community and culture that are thought to increase the likelihood that parents may abuse their children.

In contrast, secondary prevention programs assume that some parents are more at risk for child abuse than other parents. Secondary prevention efforts, which also seek to prevent child abuse prior to its occurrence, usually attempt to assess the individual risk level of parents. Parents believed to be at risk of child maltreatment are offered interventions (e.g., parenting education, parent support groups, in-home visitation) that are designed to reduce child maltreatment risk.

Tertiary prevention efforts involve intervention after the occurrence of child maltreatment (e.g., legal intervention, therapy). These interventions attempt to prevent recidivism. As in secondary prevention, risk assessment is usually an important part of tertiary intervention. As previously noted, risk assessment is a necessary part of screening reported cases. After the confirmation of maltreatment, risk assessment is important in the determination of whether a child should be removed or returned to the parent. Risk assessment also is important in the determination of treatment effects and the prediction of posttreatment recidivism, and therefore is a major part of tertiary prevention efforts.

This section has discussed the three traditional forms of intervention that attempt to reduce risk factors for child maltreatment and the associated need (or lack of need) for risk assessment within each intervention approach. It should be mentioned that there are variations on these approaches. For example, there are interventions based on developing individual/community strengths, as opposed to focusing on risk factors. In strength-based approaches, the goal is to strengthen factors that are believed to buffer or reduce the occurrence of child maltreatment. Thus, as a form of primary prevention, strength-based approaches do not screen for individual risk because the focus is not on high-risk individuals and the interventions are available community-wide to all parents.

CHILD PHYSICAL ABUSE MODELS

Ideally, risk factors assessed in secondary and tertiary prevention programs are determined by the child maltreatment models that guide the programs. Explanatory models of child maltreatment have included constructs from a variety of domains, including individual, family, community, and cultural factors. Factors in each domain are believed to have either risk potentiating or protective influences that may be transient or enduring in their effects on child abuse risk (e.g., Cicchetti & Rizley, 1981). Organizational models have described these domains as representing different ecological levels of influence (e.g., Belsky, 1980, 1993; Luster & Okagaki, 2005).

For example, Belsky (1980) described four ecological levels that may be found in etiologic models of child maltreatment; the ontogenic, microsystem, ecosystem, and macrosystem levels. The ontogenic level refers to individual factors in child abuse. At this ecological level, child abuse models focus on parent characteristics. The microsystem level refers to family factors. At this ecological level, models target factors such as parent-child interactions, marital discord, and the quality of family relations (e.g., adaptability, cohesion). At the ecosystem (community) and macrosystem (culture) levels, models include factors such as social support, unemployment stress, and cultural values. In an extension of his organizational model, Belsky (1993) described in greater detail the various "contexts of maltreatment," which include the immediate context (the parent-child interaction) and broader contexts (community, cultural, and evolutionary conditions) thought to influence the likelihood of child maltreatment.

Within the broad context of Belsky's (1980, 1993) organizational model, a large number of more specific etiological child physical abuse models have been developed, and most include factors from several, but not all, ecological levels. For example, at the beginning of the last decade, Tzeng, Jackson, and Karlson (1991) described 25 models of child physical abuse that had been generated representing nine different paradigms (e.g., sociocultural, family system, and learning paradigms). Recent model developments have focused on the refinement of extant models, such as detailed attempts to understand different aspects of social information processing in high-risk and physically abusive parents (e.g., Azar, 1997; Milner, 1993, 2000, 2003).

CHILD PHYSICAL ABUSE RISK FACTORS

As with child physical abuse models, risk assessment procedures may target a single factor at any ecological level or can be multidimensional and assess multiple factors at different ecological levels. Reviews are available that provide detailed descriptions of risk and protective factors at the individual (e.g., Milner, 1998; Milner & Dopke, 1997; Vondra, Sysko, & Belsky, 2005), family (e.g., Milner, 1998), community, and societal (e.g., Tolan & Guerra, 1998) levels.

The primary focus of this chapter is on child physical abuse risk assessment at the ontogenic (parent) and microsystem (family) levels. In practice these are the levels that typically receive professional assessment to determine individual risk even though community and cultural factors may contribute to a specific individual's risk for child abuse. Research has generally supported the use of individual and familial risk factors to predict abuse. For example, a 17-year prospective study found that as the number of individual and familial risk factors increased so did the prevalence of child abuse and neglect (from 3% when no risk factors were present to 24% when four or more risk factors were present), albeit different patterns of factors were found for child physical abuse and child neglect (Brown, Cohen, Johnson, & Salzinger, 1998).

Individual Risk Factors

At the individual level, child physical abuse risk factors can be grouped into overlapping domains of demographic/social, biological, cognitive/affective, and behavioral characteristics (e.g., see Azar & Wolfe, 2006; Milner, 1998; Milner & Dopke, 1997; for reviews).

Examples of demographic and social risk factors include: nonbiological parent, single parent, young parent, lower levels of education, large number of children, unemployment, social isolation, and a parent's childhood history of receipt and observation of maltreatment.

Putative biological risk factors include neuropsychological, psychophysiological, and physical health problems. It has been suggested that some disorders (e.g., episodic dyscontrol, attention deficit disorders), which are associated with neuropsychological deficits, are associated with child abuse. Further, it has been suggested that specific cognitive deficits, such as problems in verbal processing, reduce the parents' ability to cope with family problems, which increases the risk for child abuse. Supporting these contentions, one study found that high-risk (compared to low-risk) parents had more cognitive deficits, as assessed by neuropsychological measures. However, after risk group differences in depression and anxiety were statistically controlled, cognitive differences were no longer significant; so it is unknown whether the cognitive deficits or the negative affect, or even a common "third" variable, is the causal risk factor.

Child physical abusers are believed to possess a hyperreactive trait and to be hyperresponsive to stimuli. Although the data are not always consistent, psychophysiological studies generally support the view that abusers and at-risk parents are more physiologically reactive to stressful child and stressful non-child-related stimuli. Finally, several authors have found that child physical abusers report more physical disabilities and health problems and others have reported that abusers have more psychosomatic illness. Although it is unclear whether abusive parents have more physical health problems or simply report more physical problems, it does appear that parental reports of frequent physical health problems are associated with an increased risk for child abuse.

Cognitive and affective risk factors represent a broad array of parental personality characteristics. These factors include poor ego strength and low self-esteem, and external locus of control, which includes blaming others for one's problems. Parental cognitive risk factors include inappropriate expectations of children's behavior, negative perceptions and evaluations of children's behavior, and "misattributions" of children's responsibility for behavior, including attributions of hostile intent. In general, affective risk factors include emotions that represent negative affectivity (e.g., distress, frustration, depression, loneliness, anxiety, and anger). Further, although most child physical abusers are not mentally ill, many types of psychopathology appear to increase the risk of parenting problems, including child abuse.

With respect to behavioral risk factors, abusive parents engage in fewer interactions with their children. However, when abusers do interact they more frequently engage in negative parenting behaviors. Abusive parents use more harsh disciplinary strategies, including verbal and physical assault. In addition, abusive parents use less reasoning and explaining, as well as less praise and fewer rewards, and they are more inconsistent when they do provide praise and rewards for prosocial child behavior. Abusive parents also are more likely to have infants who have attachment problems. Beyond child-related interactional problems, abusers exhibit adult interactional problems, often displaying inadequate interpersonal skills and adult attachment problems. They often report a general inability to cope with life stress. Finally, although the frequency is debated, abusive and high-risk parents often have alcohol and drug problems.

Familial Risk Factors

Familial risk factors for child physical abuse overlap with many of the aforementioned individual risk factors. Familial demographic characteristics, such as the lack of resources and a large number of family members in an inadequate living environment, are risk factors. As the total number of stressors experienced by family members increases, so does the risk for child abuse. Frequent marital discord, including spousal abuse, is a risk factor for child physical abuse. Like marital discord, high levels of family verbal and physical conflict and social isolation, as well as the lack of family cohesion and expressiveness, are factors that increase risk.

RESEARCH ISSUES THAT IMPACT CHILD PHYSICAL ABUSE RISK ASSESSMENT

Although the literature is replete with studies describing child abuse risk factors, a major problem that limits our ability to describe and predict child physical abuse is the way the term *child physical abuse* has been operationalized. Initially child maltreatment was not carefully divided into subtypes. Even today, when child physical abuse is separated from child neglect for research purposes, child physical abuse cases may or may not exclude sexual and/or emotional child abuse. As part of the need to consider the specific types (and combinations) of child maltreatment, the study of different forms of each type, as well as whether the case is situational or chronic, appears warranted.

For example, parents who impulsively spank their children and produce mild bruises may be psychologically different from parents who intentionally burn their children. Because most descriptive and predictive child physical abuse research has been based on poorly defined groups, study results can be difficult to replicate. This difficulty adds to the likelihood of classification errors (false-positive and false-negative classifications) when attempts are made to use study findings describing risk factors to determine risk potential for a specific type of abuse.

Other problems in child physical abuse research contribute to the likelihood of classification errors. Often matched comparison groups are not used, so it is impossible to determine the extent to which group differences are due to the occurrence of child abuse or to group demographic differences (e.g., gender, ethnic background, age, educational level). In addition, cross-validation research using an array of participants is needed because abuse-related factors may be found for parents from one population (mother, Caucasian, lower Socioeconomic Status (SES) but not for parents from a demographically different population. We also do not know the extent to which the risk factors for abuse by biological parents are the same as those for abuse by nonbiological caretakers.

Even if concise definitions of child physical abuse and appropriate study designs are used, research problems remain because the existence of abuse must be indicated by some criterion, which is often the protective services worker's judgment. Unfortunately there is always the likelihood of attenuation (errors) in this and other child physical abuse criteria. Further, because protective services cases frequently are used in research, child abuse cases that are not reported are not studied. Indeed most studies include only volunteer participants, which further limits the representativeness of the results. In addition, most studies use self-report maternal data (thus, little is known about paternal risk factors), and most studies do not control for response distortions, which can be a significant problem (see Bennett, Sullivan, & Lewis, 2006; Milner & Crouch, 1997). Finally, most studies investigate and report group differences but do not report individual prediction (hit) rates for risk criteria.

DETERMINATION AND PREDICTION
OF CHILD PHYSICAL ABUSE

In child physical abuse cases, when the practitioner investigates a reported case, assessment data are often collected through relatively unstructured interviews with the victim, the suspected perpetrator, other family members, and collaterals. Unfortunately, in clinical practice, interviews can be inefficient and often provide only a limited amount of data. Unstructured procedures have been criticized for producing risk evaluations that are inconsistent and lacking accountability because of the vague or invisible criteria used in determining risk.

Interviews

Ammerman and Hersen (1999b) have pointed out that, in the assessment of family violence, interviews tend to be biased and are affected by respondent distortions and recall problems. In an attempt to guide professionals in their interviews of violent families, a number of checklists (e.g., Ayoub & Jacewitz, 1982; Murphy, Orkow, & Nicola, 1985), risk indicators (e.g., Dalgleish & Drew, 1989; Korfmacher, 2000), and interviews (e.g., Child Abuse and Neglect Interview Schedule [Ammerman, Hersen, & Van Hasselt, 1988], Parent Interview and Assessment Guide [Wolfe, 1988]) have been developed.

A major problem with existing clinical interview criteria is that each criterion lacks selectivity; that is, many (and frequently the majority of) parents exhibiting one or more of the at-risk criteria will not be abusive, resulting in an excessive number of false positive classifications. Further, child physical abuse often appears to be the result of the interaction of several contributing factors that occur in the absence of buffering conditions (factors that serve to decrease the likelihood of child maltreatment). Checklists and structured interviews typically do not provide information about which factors or group of factors provides the best prediction of child abuse, and the role of buffering variables usually is ignored.

In fairness to the authors of checklists and structured interviews, buffering variables may be excluded from risk assessment criteria because the role of buffering variables has not been fully explicated in the research literature. For example, family support and peer support appear to be important factors in reducing child physical abuse risk (e.g., Crouch, Milner, & Caliso, 1995; Crouch, Milner, & Thomsen, 2001; Egeland, Jacobvitz, & Sroufe, 1988; Milner, Robertson, & Rogers, 1990), but the specific buffering effects of different types of family and peer support on various risk factors have not been adequately determined.

It should be noted that even though checklists and structured interviews are available for assessing different types of family violence, relatively few of these instruments have any published validity data. Even when validity data are available, individual classification rates (correct classifications of abusers and comparison parents and false-positive and false-negative classifications) are rarely available. Although there are few data on the individual concurrent prediction rates of checklists and structured interviews, there are even fewer data on the future prediction of child abuse in the offender, including recidivism prediction. Finally, even if a particular structured interview can be shown to have adequate psychometric characteristics, the utility of the interview procedure still will vary as a function of the experience and skill of the interviewer.

Personality Measures

In addition to the use of checklists and structured interviews, general personality measures have been used to assess child abuse risk. In most assessment situations, it is believed that questionnaires account for a larger portion of the variance than checklist and interview procedures. Historically, the questionnaire approach has been viewed as superior to interview techniques because questionnaire data replicate and extend the information typically obtained through interviews and because questionnaires are usually less time-consuming and more economical than interviews (e.g., Nunnally, 1978).

Research on the use of existing personality measures to assess child abuse risk, however, has yielded mixed results. For example, the Minnesota Multiphasic Personality Inventory (MMPI) (Hathaway & McKinley, 1943) and the MMPI-2 (Butcher & Williams, 1992; Duckworth & Anderson, 1995), a general measure of psychopathology, has been used to distinguish abusers from nonabusers. Although the MMPI initially was believed to have utility in child abuse screening, the successful replication of MMPI profiles that were first believed to discriminate between child abusers and nonabusers has met with only limited success (e.g., Gabinet, 1979; Griswold & Billingsley, 1969; Paulson, Afifi, Chaleff, Thomason, & Liu, 1975; Paulson, Afifi, Thomason, & Chaleff, 1974).

Perhaps because of the lack of support for use of the MMPI in child physical abuse screening, with only a few exceptions (e.g., Egeland, Erickson, Butcher, & Ben-Porath, 1991), new research in the past two decades has not been forthcoming on the utility of using the MMPI to identify child physical abusers. Projective measures of personality also have been used to distinguish abusers from nonabusers. Only a few studies, however, have reported data on the effectiveness of this application (e.g., Rorschach Inkblot Test [Cyrulnik, 2000; Derr, 1978; Lerner, 1975]), and at present the extent to which projective tests have utility in the determination of individual risk for child physical abuse has not been adequately determined.

Child Physical Abuse Risk Measures

As a response to the limitations of using general personality measures to assess child physical abuse risk, a large number of measures have been developed for the specific purpose of assessing child physical abuse risk. At present, however, most of these measures do not have adequate reliability and validity data to support their use. For example, only two measures (the Michigan Screening Profile of Parenting [MSPP; Helfer, Hoffmeister, & Schneider, 1978] and the Child Abuse Potential [CAP] Inventory [Milner, 1986b, 1994, 2004]) have published validation and cross-validation data on individual (concurrent) classification rates, and only one measure (i.e., the CAP Inventory) has multiple studies reporting individual (offender) future (prospective) predictive validity data and has supportive prospective data across ethnic groups.

In situations in which current and future risk (whether immediate future risk, sometimes called safety assessment, or long-term future risk) status is a concern, supportive individual concurrent and future predictive validity data, along with cross-validation data on different populations, are needed. In the following section, psychometric data on the aforementioned CAP Inventory, one of the most commonly used child physical abuse assessment instruments, are reviewed.

The Child Abuse Potential (CAP) Inventory

The initial development of the CAP Inventory is described in a comprehensive technical manual (Milner, 1986b). An interpretive manual for the CAP Inventory scales is available as a supplement to the technical manual (Milner, 2006). Separate from material in the CAP manuals, articles on psychometric characteristics of the CAP Inventory (e.g., Milner, 1994, 2004) and on the applications and limitations of the CAP Inventory are available (Melton & Limber, 1989; Milner, 1986a, 1986b, 1989b, 1989c, 1991a, 2004, 2006).

The CAP Inventory initially was designed for use in child protective services settings to screen parents reported for child physical abuse. The questionnaire was developed because of the frequent need for additional objective information regarding a child physical abuse report. The development of a screening questionnaire for reported child physical abuse cases was viewed as appropriate because abuse base rates in reported cases of child physical abuse range from 30% to 50% in most protective services settings. A base rate near 50% is optimal for a test instrument to produce maximal increases in incremental validity. When base rates of occurrence are low, the utility of using a screening instrument is reduced. If base rates are very low (e.g., 5% or 10%), most single-test applications will not provide any meaningful increase in prediction. In such cases some form of multiple stage screening should be used to raise the base rate at each screening stage.

The CAP Inventory is a 160-item, self-report questionnaire that is answered in a forced-choice, agree-disagree format. The current CAP Inventory (Form VI) contains a 77-item child physical abuse scale that includes six descriptive factor scales: distress, rigidity, unhappiness, problems with child and self, problems with family, and problems from others. To detect response distortions, the CAP Inventory contains three validity scales: a lie scale, a random response scale, and an inconsistency scale. The validity scales are used in paired combinations to form three validity indexes: the faking-good index, the faking-bad index, and the random response index. If a response distortion index is elevated, the abuse scale scores may not be an accurate representation of the respondent's "true" score.

The applied manual for the CAP Inventory (Milner, 2006; also see Milner & Crouch, 1997) provides an extensive discussion of how the validity indexes should be interpreted. Two special scales are part of the CAP Inventory: the ego-strength scale (Milner, 1988, 2006) and the loneliness scale (Mazzucco, Gordon, & Milner, 1989; Milner, 2006). These special scales were developed from existing scale and filler items and were designed to provide the test user with supplemental clinical information on the respondent.

Concurrent Prediction of Child Physical Abuse

Initial abuse scale classification rates based on discriminant analysis for child physical abusers and matched comparison participants indicated correct classification rates in the 90% range. In subsequent studies in which more diverse populations have been used, the individual correct classification rates, again based on discriminant analysis, have been in the mid-80% to the low 90% range (e.g., Caliso & Milner, 1992; Milner, Gold, & Wimberley, 1986; Milner & Robertson, 1989).

Because discriminant analysis provides optimal classification rates for the sample under investigation, other studies have investigated CAP Inventory abuse scale classification rates determined by the standard scoring procedure. For example, in one study Milner (1989a) found that 81.4% of the abusers and 99.0% of the comparison parents were classified correctly, for an overall rate of 90.2%. Typically, in studies in which the abuse scale classification rates have been determined using the standard scoring procedure, the rates are lower than those found using discriminant analysis. Further, in studies using child physical abusers and matched comparison participants, more false negative than false positive classifications have been reported. This outcome suggests it is more likely that the abuse scale will fail to detect abusive parents (false negatives) than to misclassify demographically similar nonabusive comparison parents as abusive (false positives).

The CAP Inventory abuse scale specificity (ability to correctly classify nonabusive parents) has been investigated in a variety of nonabusive groups with acceptable results. For example, 100% correct classification rates have been reported for low-risk mothers (Lamphear, Stets, Whitaker, & Ross, 1985), nurturing mothers (Milner, 1986b, 1989a), and nurturing foster parents (Couron, 1982). In a major study ($N = 1,151$) of the effects of medical stressors on the abuse scale specificity, no distortions in specificity were found in mothers with vaginal and C-section delivery, with and without complications (Milner, 1991b). However, modest distortions in abuse scale specificity were found when parents of children with specific types of child injury (e.g., severe burns) and illness (e.g., gastric problems) were tested. Although it is possible that distortions in the abuse scale specificity may have been due to undetected child abuse, these data suggest the abuse scale specificity may be affected to some degree by a parent having a child with medical problems (Milner, 1991b). Thus, although it appears the abuse scale can be used with mothers of newborns, additional data are needed to determine whether use of the abuse scale in a medical setting with parents of children who have injuries or illness is appropriate.

In general, when abuse scale classification rates have been determined for maltreatment groups other than recently identified, untreated child physical abusers, the classification rates have been lower. For example, Matthews (1985) investigated CAP abuse scale classification rates for "mildly" abusive parents and comparison parents. To provide a stringent test of the abuse scale classification rates, the mild child physical abuse group excluded moderate and severe child physical abusers. In addition, the comparison parents had children with emotional and behavioral problems. Another sample restriction was that both parent groups already were receiving treatment. Using a cutoff score developed from half of the study sample, Matthews (1985) reported a correct CAP abuse scale classification rate of 72.7%.

Couron (1982) studied a physically abusive and neglectful parent group (even though the abuse scale was not designed to detect neglectful parents) and a comparison parent group and found that when the abuse scale alone was used to predict group membership, the correct classification rate was 72.6%. A discriminant analysis, however, indicated an overall correct classification rate of 90.3% when the abuse score, a stress measure, and demographic characteristics (e.g., marital status, age of parent) were used to predict group membership.

In another study, Haddock and McQueen (1983) reported abuse scale classification rates for institutional child physical abusers and matched nonabusive institutional employees. A discriminant analysis indicated an overall correct classification rate of 92.9% by using the CAP abuse scale, work satisfaction items, and demographic variables to predict group membership. Although this overall classification rate for institutional abusers is encouraging, the institutional abuser classification rate for the CAP abuse scale alone was not reported.

Collectively these data suggest the CAP abuse scale may have some validity when used as a screening tool with groups other than suspected child physical abusers who are investigated by social services agencies. However, because the CAP abuse scale was designed for use with parents, additional data (e.g., individual classification rates) are needed to determine the extent to which the CAP abuse scale can be used with different nonparent groups.

Finally, the CAP Inventory has been translated into more than 25 languages with varying degrees of cross-validation research having been completed on these translated versions. Spanish translations have been the most frequently studied translations. Correct (concurrent) classification rates similar to those found for the English version have been reported for different Spanish translations of the CAP Inventory abuse scale using child physical abusers and comparison parents in Spain (De Paul, Arruabarrena, & Milner, 1991, 1998a, 1998b; De Paul, Arruabarrena, Múgica, & Milner, 1999), in Argentina (Barbich & Bringiotti, 1997; Bringiotti, Barbich, & De Paul, 1998), and in Chile (Calderón et al., 1994; Haz & Ramirez, 1998; but see Haz & Ramirez, 2002, for an exception).

Future Prediction of Child Maltreatment

In addition to concurrent validity data, longitudinal predictive validity data are available for the CAP abuse scale. Milner, Gold, Ayoub, and Jacewitz (1984) found a significant ($p < .0001$) relationship between elevated abuse scores and later child physical abuse in a group of at-risk parents who were in treatment ($\omega^2 = .32$). A modest relationship ($p < .05$) was found between abuse scores and later child neglect.

In another study, Ayoub and Milner (1985) found that abuse scores of mothers of failure-to-thrive infants receiving services were significantly ($p < .01$) related to later instances of child neglect. In another prospective study that followed 1,488 parents or expectant parents recruited from 28 family support or family preservation programs, Valle, Chaffin, and BigFoot (2000) reported abuse scores taken when parents entered the programs predicted later incidences of child maltreatment (after controlling for demographic factors). Additional analyses indicated abuse scores predicted future child maltreatment in Caucasian, Native American, and African American participants but showed only a trend in Hispanic participants. In another study by two of the same authors in what appears to be a subset of the same parents, posttreatment abuse scores were not found to be associated with later abuse (Chaffin & Valle, 2003). However, it is unclear if the lack of prediction was due to the inability of the abuse scale to predict following treatment or if the abuse scale reductions posttreatment were accurate at that point in time but were not predictive of later abuse because the treatment effects were only temporary.

Several prospective studies report of the relationship between maternal CAP abuse scores and negative child outcomes other than child maltreatment. For example, Dukewich, Borkowski, and Whitman (1999) reported maternal CAP abuse scores obtained when their children were 1 and 3 years of age were predictive of their children's adaptive behavior and intelligence at 3 and 5 years of age. The maternal CAP abuse scores' prediction of children's later developmental problems remained significant after maternal problematic parenting orientations were statistically controlled. Zelenko et al. (2001) examined the relationship between prenatal maternal CAP abuse scores (on a shortened version of the CAP abuse scale) and neonatal morbidity. Prenatal maternal abuse scores were significant predictors of neonatal morbidity and this association remained significant even after obstetric risk factors were statistically controlled.

Although in all studies reviewed the total CAP abuse score has been superior to the individual factor scores in predicting abuse, the predictive validity data indicate that some abuse factor scales are better at predicting concurrent risk and that others are better at predicting future risk. For example, the level of parent-child-related distress factor scale appears to be a strong predictor of concurrent risk, whereas a rigid pattern of expectations of child behavior factor scale appears to be a relatively better predictor of future abuse, even though both factors significantly predict concurrent and future child physical abuse. This finding may be related to the distress factor's tendency to measure situational conditions that change across time, whereas the rigidity factor appears to measure trait-like conditions that are less likely to change across time. Thus, on the basis of the type of prediction desired, the test user may want to consider the extent to which the different factor scores are elevated.

Construct Validity

A representative, albeit not exhaustive, list of the CAP Inventory abuse scale construct validity studies by domain is provided in this section.[2]

The construct validity research indicates that the individual child physical abuse risk factors discussed previously are related generally to CAP abuse scores in the expected manner. For example, individuals with childhood histories of physical abuse tend to earn higher abuse scores than individuals without such histories. In general, individuals with elevated abuse scores report more family conflict, less family cohesion, and more social isolation. When supportive relationships (adult or peer) occur during childhood, however, the abuse scores reflect these buffering events and tend to be lower.

Although it is unclear if individuals with elevated abuse scores are more likely to have an insecurely attached infant, they do display insecure adult attachments. An inverse relationship has been observed between abuse scores and self-esteem and ego-strength. Persons with elevated abuse scores also tend to have an external locus of control. Elevated abuse scores appear to be related to at least two types of external control orientations: control by chance factors and control by powerful others.

As expected, elevated abuse scores have been associated with higher levels of life stress and personal distress. Further, individuals with elevated abuse scores tend to be more physiologically reactive to both child-related and non-child-related stimuli and display neuropsychological deficits. Those with elevated abuse scores report more negative perceptions of their children's behavior and are more critical and less praising of their children. Parents with elevated abuse scores display a rigid interactional style and are less responsive to temporal changes in their children's behavior. They make more negative interpretations and evaluations of their children's behavior, use more verbal and physical punishment, react to children in a controlling and rejecting manner, and are less likely to respond consistently to prosocial behaviors. Elevated abuse scores and stress interact, increasing the parent's aversive, child-directed behaviors. Given these findings, it is not surprising that parents with elevated abuse scores report less satisfaction with the quality of their child attachments.

Additional research indicates individuals with elevated abuse scores tend to be depressed, moody, touchy, emotionally labile, overreactive, and aggressive. Similarly those with elevated abuse scores have been described as lacking emotional stability, having a low frustration tolerance, being irritable, having poor impulse control, having temper outbursts, being assaultive, and displaying less empathy. Elevated abuse scores also are correlated with alcohol and drug use.

Although individual classification rates are not always adequate, studies of child maltreatment groups other than child physical abusers indicate the abuse scale distinguishes groups in the expected manner. For example, the abuse scale discriminates between groups of at-risk and comparison participants and between groups thought to differ in levels of risk. Abuse scores have distinguished between institutional child abusers and a nonabusive comparison (employee) group and among child physical abusers, intrafamilial sexual child abusers, child neglecters, and three matched comparison groups. Because of common perpetrator characteristics, however, the abuse scale did not adequately discriminate between the different child maltreatment groups.

A number of studies have reported abuse score decreases after intervention. For example, pretreatment, posttreatment, and follow-up abuse score decreases have been reported for at-risk parents presented an ecologically based intervention program. Pretreatment and follow-up abuse score decreases have been found for at-risk parents given a behavioral parent training program. Pre- and posttreatment abuse score decreases have been reported for a group of abusive and neglectful parents after an intensive multimodal intervention program. Several studies have reported abuse score decreases after in-home treatments. Finally, initial (very high) abuse scores have been reported to be predictors of client dropout. Collectively the treatment evaluation studies indicate the CAP abuse scale is a useful global measure of treatment effects for at-risk and abusive parent treatment programs.

Reliability

The CAP Inventory abuse scale internal consistency (KR-20) reliabilities reported in the technical manual range from .91 to .96 for general population ($N = 2,062$), at-risk ($N = 124$), neglectful ($N = 209$), and physically abusive ($N = 149$) groups (Milner, 1986b). Similar abuse scale internal consistency estimates are reported across gender, age, education, and ethnic subgroups (Milner, 1986b). These initial internal consistency reliability estimates have been replicated in subsequent studies (e.g., Black et al., 1994; Bringiotti et al., 1998; Caliso & Milner, 1992; De Paul et al., 1991; Haz & Ramirez, 1998; Merrill, Hervig, & Milner, 1996; Milner & Robertson, 1990; Pecnik & Ajdukovic, 1995). The child physical abuse scale temporal stability (test-retest) reliabilities are .91, .90, .83, and .75 for general population participants across 1-day, 1-week, 1-month, and 3-month intervals, respectively (Milner, 1986b). Internal consistency and temporal stability estimates also are available for each of the three validity scales and the six descriptive factor scales (Milner, 1986b).

Other Measures Frequently Used in Child Physical Abuse Risk Assessment

A self-report questionnaire, which was the first "objective" scale developed to screen for child physical abuse, is the Michigan Screening Profile of Parenting (MSPP) (Helfer et al., 1978; Schneider, 1982). As a consequence of validity research, however, the authors expanded the scope of the MSPP and now recommend the scale be used for the screening of parents with problems in parenting, rather than for the screening of child physical abuse. Although the individual classification rates for child physical abusers were adequate, research indicated the MSPP has relatively high rates of false positive classifications even in nurturing parent groups (e.g., Schneider, 1982). A literature review failed to yield any additional studies on the MSPP classification rates.

A well-known self-report survey instrument that was intended to measure physical abuse, psychological maltreatment, and neglect is the Parent-Child Conflict Tactics Scale (CTSPC) (Strauss, Hamby, Finkelhor, Moore, & Runyan, 1998a, 1998b). However, Bennett et al. (2006) reported mixed results with respect to maltreatment group classifications using the CTSPC. Further, no data are available on the individual classification rates using the CTSPC to classify known abusive and matched nonabusive comparison groups.

Another self-report measure, the Parenting Stress Index (PSI) (Abidin, 1995, 1997, 2006), has been developed to assess parent and child-related stress separate from general life stress. This scale appears to be a useful measure of parenting stress and has distinguished groups of child physical abusers and comparison parents. Even though the PSI was not initially designed to screen for child physical abuse, the PSI does appear to have utility in the evaluation of dysfunctional parent-child dyads and for use in treatment planning and program evaluation (e.g., Abidin, 2006). In light of the extensive and supportive psychometric base of the PSI, it is unfortunate that data still are needed to determine the utility of using the PSI to individually classify child physical abusers.

Finally, a self-report measure, the Adult/Adolescent Parenting Inventory (AAPI), has been developed to assess parent and adolescent attitudes and expectations (Bavolek, 1984, 1989) with respect to children. As with many attitude and personality measures, the AAPI and revised AAPI-2 have been shown to distinguish between groups of child physical abusers and comparison parents and has been promoted as an at-risk screening instrument. However, the utility of the AAPI and subsequent AAPI-2 as an individual risk screening scale remains to be fully determined (e.g., Connors, Whiteside-Mansell, Deere, Ledet, & Edwards, 2006; Lutenbacher, 2001), in part, because individual classification rates based on the AAPI and AAPI-2 for child physical abusers and matched comparison parents are not available.

In addition to the aforementioned measures, a larger number of other individual and family measures have been developed that may have some utility in child abuse assessment. Reviews of child physical abuse assessment techniques are provided elsewhere (e.g., Hansen & MacMillan, 1990; Hansen & Warner, 1992; Milner, Murphy, Valle, & Tolliver, 1998). Comprehensive reviews of individual and family measures that provide information on a wide variety of problems that may occur in high-risk and abusive families also are available (e.g., Ammerman & Hersen, 1999a; Feindler, Rathus, & Silver, 2003).

Finally, because of the widespread interest in risk assessment, the National Center on Child Abuse and Neglect (NCCAN) supported the development and testing of a number of risk assessment protocols. A discussion of risk assessment problems and ongoing risk assessment research is provided in a conference proceedings (Cicchinelli, 1991) sponsored by NCCAN. Although their description is beyond the scope of this chapter, these risk assessment systems include perpetrator factors, as well as factors from each of the other ecological levels previously mentioned in the description of Belsky's (1980) ecological model. It also appears that these systems have a variety of purposes (e.g., current abuse risk versus recidivism prediction).

McDonald and Marks (1991) described and evaluated some of the major risk-assessment systems found in the field. Their review included the following assessment systems: the Alameda County California Reabuse Assessment Model, the Washington Risk Factor Matrix, the Illinois CANTS 17B, the Utah Risk Assessment Model, the Florida Health and Rehabilitation Services Child Risk Assessment Matrix, the Child Welfare League Family Risk Scales, and the Action for Child Protection Child at Risk Scales. With respect to the content of the scales, McDonald and Marks conclude, "There is little empirical support for most of the included variables," yet indicated that "subsets of variables can be identified that are common to most instruments and that have empirical support" (1991, p. 112).

Unfortunately, a search of the literature since the McDonald and Marks review 15 years ago revealed that only several studies, for example, two outcome studies (Lyle & Graham, 2000; Zeece & Wang, 1999) and one recidivism study (Camasso & Jagannathan, 1996), have been published on any of the assessment procedures covered in the McDonald and Marks review. The recidivism study evaluated the Washington State Risk Matrix and the Illinois CANTS 17B, using protective services cases. Regression analyses revealed that both procedures predicted case recidivism better than chance but additional data are needed to determine their potential utility in individual classification. Further, there is a need to compare assessments by using these systems with other forms of assessment (e.g., questionnaires) and to determine the utility of using these systems in combination with other approaches.

SUMMARY

An array of adult risk characteristics for child physical abuse have been identified that can be used to guide risk assessment. However, not all clients will have these characteristics, and it is not clear which risk characteristics, or combinations of risk characteristics, are the best predictors of child physical abuse. Further, the available risk assessment techniques (e.g., structured interviews, tests) have varying degrees of reliability and validity. Test users must remember that a measure may have adequate validity for one particular application (e.g., program evaluation) with one population (e.g., adult parents) and not be appropriate for another application (e.g., future prediction) with another population (e.g., adolescent mothers). At present it appears the best overall risk prediction can be obtained when risk assessment includes data on multiple risk factors from as many sources as possible, include structured parent interviews, collateral interviews, direct observations, and testing with multiple objective measures. When risk factors appear across data sources, the factors can be used to make an estimate of overall risk, with an awareness that mistakes in risk assessment still will occur, especially in situations in which abuse rates are low in the population under investigation.

NOTES

1. Although the number of official cases reported by child protective services (CPS) agencies remains alarmingly high, survey research supports the view that the majority of child maltreatment cases are never referred to child protective services. For example, in a national incidence study of child abuse and neglect, only 28% of child maltreatment events found in the national survey that meet criteria for child maltreatment had been referred to CPS (Sedlak & Broadhurst, 1996).
2. The construct validity data reported in this section are based on more than 100 studies. Due to space limitations, individual citations are not provided in this chapter. However, upon request the author will provide (pro bono) a reading list of more than 500 papers, studies, chapters, theses, dissertations, unpublished works, and so forth on the uses and psychometric characteristics of the CAP Inventory, which include citations documenting the degree to which the CAP Inventory abuse scale is associated with each of the constructs discussed in this chapter.

REFERENCES

Abidin, R. R. (1995). *Parenting Stress Index: Manual* (3rd ed.). Odessa, FL: Psychological Assessment Resources.

Abidin, R. R. (1997). Parenting Stress Index: A measure of the parent-child system. In C. P. Zalaquett & R. L. Wood (Eds.), *Evaluating stress: A book of resources* (pp. 277–291). Lanham, MD: Scarecrow Press.

Abidin, R. R. (2006). The Parenting Stress Index. In R. P. Archer (Ed.), *Forensic uses of clinical assessment instruments* (pp. 297–328). Mahwah, NJ: Lawrence Erlbaum Associates Publishers.

Ammerman, R. T., & Hersen, M. (Eds.) (1999a). *Assessment of family violence: A clinical and legal sourcebook.* New York: John Wiley.

Ammerman, R. T., & Hersen, M. (1999b). Current issues in the assessment of family violence: An update. In R. T. Ammerman & M. Hersen (Eds.), *Assessment of family violence: A clinical and legal sourcebook* (pp. 3–9). New York: John Wiley.

Ammerman, R. T., Hersen, M., & Van Hasselt, V. B. (1988). *The Child Abuse and Neglect Interview Schedule (CANTS)*. Unpublished instrument, Western Pennsylvania School for Blind Children, Pittsburgh.

Ayoub, C., & Jacewitz, M. M. (1982). Families at risk of poor parenting: A model for service delivery, assessment, and intervention. *Child Abuse & Neglect, 6,* 351–358.

Ayoub, C., & Milner, J. S. (1985). Failure-to-thrive: Parental indicators, types, and outcomes. *Child Abuse & Neglect, 9,* 491–499.

Azar, S. T. (1997). A cognitive behavioral approach to understanding and treating parents who physically abuse their children. In D. A. Wolfe, R. J. McMahon, & R. deV. Peters (Eds.), *Child abuse: New directions in prevention and treatment across the life span* (pp. 79–101). Thousand Oaks, CA: Sage.

Azar, S. T., & Wolfe, D. A. (2006). Child physical abuse and neglect. In E. J. Mash & R. A. Barkley (Eds.), *Treatment of childhood disorders* (3rd ed.), (pp. 595–646). New York: Guilford Press.

Barbich, A., & Bringiotti, M. I. (1997). Un estudio para la adaptación y validación del CAP (Child Abuse Potential Inventory) para su uso en la Argentina. *Revista del Instituto de Investigaciones de la Facultad de Psicología, 2*(2), 15–31.

Bavolek, S. J. (1984). *Adult-Adolescent Parenting Inventory (AAPI)*. Eau Claire, WI: Family Development Resources.

Bavolek, S. J. (1989). Assessing and treating high-risk parenting attitudes. In J. T. Pardeck (Ed.), *Child abuse and neglect: Theory, research, and practice* (pp. 97–110). New York: Gordon & Breach.

Belsky, J. (1980). Child maltreatment: An ecological integration. *American Psychologist, 35,* 320–335.

Belsky, J. (1993). Etiology of child maltreatment: A developmental-ecological analysis. *Psychological Bulletin, 114,* 413–434.

Bennett, D. S., Sullivan, M. W., & Lewis, M. (2006). Relations of parental report and observation of parenting to maltreatment history. *Child Maltreatment, 11,* 63–75.

Black, M. M., Nair, P., Kight, C., Wachtel, R., Roby, P., & Schuler, M. (1994). Parenting and early development among children of drug-abusing women: Effects of home intervention. *Pediatrics, 94,* 440–448.

Bringiotti, M. I., Barbich, A., & De Paul, J. (1998). Validación de una versión preliminar del Child Abuse Potential Inventory para su uso en Argentina. *Child Abuse & Neglect, 22,* 881–888.

Brown, J., Cohen, P., Johnson, J. G., & Salzinger, S. (1998). A longitudinal analysis of risk factors for child maltreatment: Findings of a 17-year prospective study of officially recorded and self-reported child abuse and neglect. *Child Abuse & Neglect, 22,* 1065–1978.

Butcher, J. N., & Williams, C. L. (1992). *Essentials of MMPI-2 and MMPI-A interpretation*. Minneapolis: University of Minnesota Press.

Calderón, V., Muñoz, D., Valdebenito, L., Fontecilla, I. M., Larrain, S., & Wenk, E. (1994). *Validación de una versión preliminar Chilena del Child Abuse Potential Inventory para su uso en Chile*. Unpublished manuscript, Facultad de Ciencias Sociales, Universidad de Chile, Santiago.

Caliso, J. A., & Milner, J. S. (1992). Childhood history of abuse and child abuse screening. *Child Abuse & Neglect, 16,* 647–659.

Camasso, M. J., & Jagannathan, R. (1996). Prediction accuracy of the Washington and Illinois risk assessment instruments: An application of receiver operating characteristics curve analyses. *Social Work Research, 19,* 174–183.

Chaffin, M., & Valle, L. A. (2003). Dynamic prediction characteristics of the Child Abuse Potential Inventory. *Child Abuse & Neglect, 27,* 463–481.

Cicchetti, D., & Rizley, R. (1981). Developmental perspectives on the etiology, intergenerational transmission, and sequelae of child maltreatment. In R. Rizley & D. Cicchetti (Eds.), *Developmental perspectives on child maltreatment* (pp. 31–55). San Francisco: Jossey-Bass.

Cicchinelli, L. F. (Ed.) (1991). *Proceedings of a symposium on risk assessment in child protective services.* Washington, DC: National Center on Child Abuse and Neglect.

Connors, N. A., Whiteside-Mansell, L., Deere, D., Ledet, T., & Edwards, M. C. (2006). Measuring the potential for child maltreatment: The reliability and validity of the Adult Adolescent Parenting Inventory-2. *Child Abuse & Neglect, 30,* 39–53,

Couron, B. L. (1982). Assessing parental potentials for child abuse in contrast to nurturing (Doctoral dissertation, United States International University, 1981). *Dissertation Abstracts International, 43,* 3412.

Crouch, J. L., Milner, J. S., & Caliso, J. A. (1995). Childhood physical abuse, perceived social support, and socio-emotional status in adulthood. *Violence and Victims, 10,* 273–283.

Crouch, J. L., Milner, J. S., & Thomsen, C. (2001). Childhood physical abuse, early social support, and risk for maltreatment: Current support as a mediator of risk for child physical abuse. *Child Abuse & Neglect, 25,* 93–107.

Cyrulnik, J. (2000). Aggressive responses in Rorschach protocols of women accused of physical child abuse and neglect (Doctoral dissertation, Miami Institute of the Caribbean Center for Advanced Studies, 2000). *Dissertation Abstracts International, 61,* 2812.

Dalgleish, L. I., & Drew, E. C. (1989). The relationship of child abuse indicators to the assessment of perceived risk and to the court's decision to separate. *Child Abuse & Neglect, 13,* 491–506.

De Paul, J., Arruabarrena, M. I., & Milner, J. S. (1991). Validación de una versión española del Child Abuse Potential Inventory para su uso en España. *Child Abuse & Neglect, 15,* 495–504.

De Paul, J., Arruabarrena, M. I., & Milner, J. S. (1998a). *CAPTEST: Manual para la corrección informatizada del Inventario de Potencial de Maltrato Infantil.* San Sebastián, España: Librería Zorroaga.

De Paul, J., Arruabarrena, M. I., & Milner, J. S. (1998b). *Manual de utilización e interpretación: Inventario de Potencial de Maltrato Infantil (CAP).* San Sebastián, España: Librería Zorroaga.

De Paul, J., Arruabarrena, M. I., Múgica, P., & Milner, J. S. (1999). Validación Española del Child Abuse Potential Inventory. *Estudios de Psicología, 62–63,* 55–72.

Derr, J. (1978). Using the Rorschach Inkblot Test in the assessment of parents charged with child abuse and neglect. *British Journal of Projective Psychology and Personality Study, 23,* 29–31.

Duckworth, J. C., & Anderson, W. P. (1995). *MMPI & MMPI-2: Interpretation manual for counselors and clinicians* (4th ed.). Philadelphia, PA: Accelerated Development.

Dukewich, T. L., Borkowski, J. G., & Whitman, T. L. (1999). A longitudinal analysis of maternal abuse potential and development delays in children of adolescent mothers. *Child Abuse & Neglect, 23,* 405–420.

Egeland, B., Erickson, M. F., Butcher, J. N., & Ben-Porath, Y. S. (1991). MMPI-2 profiles of women at risk for child abuse. *Journal of Personality Assessment, 57,* 254–263.

Egeland, B., Jacobvitz, D., & Sroufe, L. A. (1988). Breaking the cycle of violence. *Child Development, 59,* 1080–1088.

Feindler, E. L., Rathus, J. H., & Silver, L. B. (2003). *Assessment of family violence: A handbook for researchers and practitioners.* Washington, DC: American Psychological Association.

Gabinet, L. (1979). MMPI profiles of high-risk and outpatient mothers. *Child Abuse & Neglect, 3,* 373–379.

Griswold, B. B., & Billingsley, A. (1969). *Personality and social characteristics of low-income mothers who neglect and abuse their children* (Final report, PR11001R). Washington, DC: Department of Health, Education, and Welfare, Children's Bureau.

Haddock, M. D., & McQueen, W. M. (1983). Assessing employee potentials for abuse. *Journal of Clinical Psychology, 39,* 1021–1029.

Hansen, D. J., & MacMillan, V. M. (1990). Behavioral assessment of child-abusive and neglectful families: Recent developments and current issues. *Behavior Modification, 14,* 255–278.

Hansen, D. J., & Warner, J. E. (1992). Child physical abuse and neglect. In R. T. Ammerman & M. Hersen (Eds.), *Assessment of family violence: A clinical and legal sourcebook* (pp. 123–147). New York: John Wiley.

Hathaway, S. R., & McKinley, J. C. (1943). *The Minnesota Multiphasic Personality Inventory.* Minneapolis: University of Minnesota Press.

Haz, A. M., & Ramirez, V. (1998). Preliminary validation of the Child Abuse Potential Inventory in Chile. *Child Abuse & Neglect, 22,* 869–879.

Haz, A. M., & Ramirez, V. (2002). Adaptation of the Child Abuse Potential Inventory in Chile: Analysis of the difficulties and challenges of its application in two Chilean studies. *Child Abuse & Neglect, 26,* 481–495.

Helfer, R. E., Hoffmeister, J. K., & Schneider, C. J. (1978). *MSPP: A manual for the use of the Michigan Screening Profile of Parenting.* Boulder, CO: Test Analyses and Development.

Korfmacher, J. (2000). The Kempe Family Stress Inventory: A review. *Child Abuse & Neglect, 24,* 129–140.

Lamphear, V. S., Stets, J. P., Whitaker, P., & Ross, A. O. (1985, August). *Maladjustment in at-risk for physical child abuse and behavior problem children: Differences in family environment and marital discord.* Paper presented at the meeting of the American Psychological Association, Los Angeles, CA.

Lerner, P. M. (1975). Rorschach measures of family interaction. A review. In P. M. Lerner (Ed.), *Handbook of Rorschach Scales* (pp. 55–67). New York: International University Press.

Luster, T., & Okagaki, L. (Eds.). (2005). *Parenting: An ecological perspective* (2nd ed.). Mahwah, NJ: Lawrence Erlbaum Associates.

Lutenbacher, M. (2001). Psychometric assessment of the Adult-Adolescent Parenting Inventory in a sample of low-income single mothers. *Journal of Nursing Measurement, 9,* 291–308.

Lyle, C., & Graham, E. (2000). Looks can be deceiving: Using a risk assessment instrument to evaluate the outcomes of child protective services. *Child & Youth Services Review, 22,* 935–949.

Matthews, R. D. (1985). Screening and identification of child abusing parents through self-report inventories (Doctoral dissertation, Florida Institute of Technology, 1984). *Dissertation Abstracts International, 46,* 650.

Mazzucco, M., Gordon, R. A., & Milner, J. S. (1989). *Development of a loneliness scale for the Child Abuse Potential Inventory.* Paper presented at the meeting of the Southeastern Psychological Association, Washington, DC.

McDonald, T., & Marks, J. (1991). A review of risk factors assessed in child protective services. *Social Service Review, 65,* 112–132.

Melton, G. B., & Limber, S. (1989). Psychologists' involvement in cases of child maltreatment. Limits of role and expertise. *American Psychologist, 44,* 400–411.

Merrill, L. L., Hervig, L. K., & Milner, J. S. (1996). Childhood parenting experiences, intimate partner conflict resolution, and adult risk for child physical abuse. *Child Abuse & Neglect, 20,* 1049–1065.

Milner, J. S. (1986a). Assessing child maltreatment: The role of testing. *Journal of Sociology and Social Welfare, 13,* 64–76.

Milner, J. S. (1986b). *The child abuse potential inventory: Manual* (2nd ed.). Webster, NC: Psytec.

Milner, J. S. (1988). An ego-strength scale for the Child Abuse Potential Inventory. *Journal of Family Violence, 3,* 151–162.

Milner, J. S. (1989a). Additional cross-validation of the Child Abuse Potential Inventory. *Psychological Assessment, 1,* 219–223.

Milner, J. S. (1989b). Applications and limitations of the Child Abuse Potential Inventory. *Early Child Development and Care, 42,* 85–97.

Milner, J. S. (1989c). Applications of the Child Abuse Potential Inventory. *Journal of Clinical Psychology, 45,* 450–454.

Milner, J. S. (1991a). Additional issues in child abuse assessment. *American Psychologist, 46,* 80–81.

Milner, J. S. (1991b). Medical conditions and Child Abuse Potential Inventory specificity. *Psychological Assessment, 3,* 208–212.

Milner, J. S. (1993). Social information processing and physical child abuse. *Clinical Psychology Review, 13,* 275–294.

Milner, J. S. (1994). Assessing physical child abuse risk: The Child Abuse Potential Inventory. *Clinical Psychology Review, 14,* 547–583.

Milner, J. S. (1998). Individual and family characteristics associated with intrafamilial child physical and sexual abuse. In P. K. Trickett & C. J. Schellenbach (Eds.), *Violence against children in the family and the community* (pp. 141–170). Washington, DC: American Psychological Association.

Milner, J. S. (2000). Social information processing and child physical abuse: Theory and research. In D. J. Hansen (Ed.), *Nebraska Symposium on Motivation: Vol. 45. Motivation and child maltreatment* (pp. 39–84). Lincoln, NE: University of Nebraska Press.

Milner, J. S. (2003). Social information processing in high-risk and physically abusive parents. *Child Abuse & Neglect, 27,* 7–20.

Milner, J. S. (2004). The Child Abuse Potential (CAP) Inventory. In M. J. Hilsenroth & D. L. Segal (Eds.), *Comprehensive handbook of psychological assessment: Vol. 2. Personality assessment* (pp. 237–246). Hoboken, NJ: Wiley.

Milner, J. S. (2006). *An interpretive manual for the Child Abuse Potential Inventory.* DeKalb, IL: Psytec.

Milner, J. S., & Crouch, J. L. (1997). Impact and detection of response distortions on parenting measures used to assess risk for child physical abuse. *Journal of Personality Assessment, 69,* 633–650.

Milner, J. S., & Dopke, C. (1997). Child physical abuse: Review of offender characteristics. In D. A. Wolfe, R. J. McMahon, & R. deV. Peters (Eds.), *Child abuse: New directions in prevention and treatment across the life span* (pp. 25–52). Thousand Oaks, CA: Sage Publications.

Milner, J. S., Gold, R. G., Ayoub, C., & Jacewitz, M. M. (1984). Predictive validity of the Child Abuse Potential Inventory. *Journal of Consulting and Clinical Psychology, 52,* 879–884.

Milner, J. S., Gold, R. G., & Wimberley, R. C. (1986). Prediction and explanation of child abuse: Cross-validation of the Child Abuse Potential Inventory. *Journal of Consulting and Clinical Psychology, 54,* 865–866.

Milner, J. S., Murphy, W. D., Valle, L., & Tolliver, R. M. (1998). Assessment issues in child abuse evaluations. In J. R. Lutzker (Ed.), *Handbook of child abuse research and treatment* (pp. 75–115). New York: Plenum.

Milner, J. S., & Robertson, K. R. (1989). Inconsistent response patterns and the prediction of child maltreatment. *Child Abuse & Neglect, 13,* 59–64.

Milner, J. S., & Robertson, K. R. (1990). Comparison of physical child abusers, intrafamilial sexual child abusers, and child neglecters. *Journal of Interpersonal Violence, 5,* 37–48.

Milner, J. S., Robertson, K. R., & Rogers, D. L. (1990). Childhood history of abuse and adult abuse potential. *Journal of Family Violence, 5,* 15–34.

Murphy, S., Orkow, B., & Nicola, R. (1985). Prenatal prediction of child abuse and neglect: A prospective study. *Child Abuse & Neglect, 9,* 225–235.

Nunnally, J. C. (1978). *Psychometric theory.* New York: McGraw-Hill.

Paulson, M. J., Afifi, A. A., Chaleff, A., Thomason, M. L., & Liu, V. Y. (1975). An MMPI scale for identifying "at-risk" abusive parents. *Journal of Clinical Child Psychology, 4,* 22–24.

Paulson, M. J., Afifi, A. A., Thomason, M. L., & Chaleff, A. (1974). The MMPI: A descriptive measure of psychopathology in abusive parents. *Journal of Clinical Psychology, 30,* 387–390.

Pecnik, N., & Ajdukovic, M. (1995). The Child Abuse Potential Inventory: Cross validation in Croatia. *Psychological Reports, 76,* 979–985.

Schneider, C. J. (1982). The Michigan Screening Profile of Parenting. In R. H. Starr (Ed.), *Child abuse prediction: Policy implications* (pp. 157–174). Cambridge, MA: Ballinger.

Sedlak, A. J., & Broadhurst, D. D. (1996). *Third national incidence study of child abuse and neglect.* Washington, DC: U.S. Government Printing Office.

Strauss, M. A., Hamby, S. L., Finkelhor, D., Moore, D. W., & Runyan, D. (1998a). Identification of child maltreatment with the Parent-Child Conflict Tactics Scales: Development and psychometric data for a national sample of American parents. *Child Abuse & Neglect, 22,* 249–270.

Strauss, M. A., Hamby, S. L., Finkelhor, D., Moore, D. W., & Runyan, D. (1998b). "Identification of child maltreatment with the Parent-Child Conflict Tactics Scales: Development and psychometric data for a national sample of American parents". Erratum. *Child Abuse & Neglect, 22,* 1177.

Tolan, P., & Guerra, N. (1998). Societal causes of violence against children. In P. Trickett & C. Schellenbach (Eds.), *Violence against children in the family and the community* (pp. 195–209). Washington, DC: American Psychological Association.

Tzeng, O., Jackson, J., & Karlson, H. (1991). *Theories of child abuse and neglect: Differential perspectives, summaries, and evaluations.* New York: Praeger.

U.S. Department of Health and Human Services, Administration on Children, Youth, and Families. (2006). *Child maltreatment 2004.* Washington, DC: U.S. Government Printing Office.

Valle, L. A., Chaffin, M., & BigFoot, D. S. (2000, July). *Assessing parenting risk in different ethnic groups with the Child Abuse Potential Inventory.* Paper presented at the meeting of the American Professional Society on the Abuse of Children, Chicago.

Vondra, J., Sysko, H. B., & Belsky, J. (2005). Developmental origins of parenting: Personality and relationship factors. In T. Luster & L. Okagaki (Eds.), *Parenting: An ecological perspective* (2nd ed., pp. 35–71). Mahwah, NJ: Lawrence Erlbaum Associates.

Wolfe, D. A. (1988). Child abuse and neglect. In E. J. Mash & L. G. Terdal (Eds.), *Behavioral assessment of childhood disorders* (2nd ed., pp. 627–669). New York: Guilford.

Zeece, P. D., & Wang, A. (1999). Effect of the Family Empowerment and Transitioning Program on child and family outcomes. *Child Study Journal, 28,* 161–178.

Zelenko, M. A., Huffman, L. C., Brown, B. W., Jr., Daniels, K., Lock, J., Kennedy, Q., et al. (2001). The Child Abuse Potential Inventory and pregnancy outcome in expectant adolescent mothers. *Child Abuse & Neglect, 25,* 1481–1495.

CHAPTER 4

Evaluating Risk Factors for Fatal Child Abuse

Scott D. Krugman and Richard D. Krugman

One of the earliest discussions of fatal child abuse was published in 1860 by Ambroise Tardieu, a French Professor of Legal Medicine in Paris. His classic paper, reprinted in 2005 (Roche, Fortin, Labbe, Brown, & Chadwick, 2005) described the autopsy findings of 32 child fatalities of Parisian children—19 of whom were killed by their parents. Tardieu's call for French physicians and society to do something about the problem of these child fatalities was ignored.

In 1995, Donna Shalala, then Secretary of the Department of Health and Human Services, called child abuse fatalities "the Nation's shame" (U.S. Advisory Board on Child Abuse and Neglect, 1995). Not much has been done by our federal government to ameliorate the problem, either by her in the last 5 years of her term, nor in the 6 years (at the time of this writing) by the current administration in Washington. Few events challenge our child protection system as much as the death of infants and children—whether by violent beatings or shakings, deliberate or incidental poisoning (e.g., living in a home methamphetamine lab), or as a result of neglect (either a lack of supervision or emotional neglect). The U.S. Advisory Board Report referenced above showed that many of the children fatally abused were known to the child protection system and had open cases at the time of their death.

Why does that happen? Can't we predict when a child will be subject to a fatal attack? And can't we predict who will fatally abuse or neglect an infant?

Sadly, the answer is that we cannot. While we do know some things about the prediction of who will be at risk for abusing a child (see Chapter 3), we cannot predict reliably when the abuse will occur and when it will be fatal. Given that reality, this chapter will review the forms fatal child abuse takes, the incidence of the problem, the risk factors that contribute to fatalities, the approaches we can take as a society to reduce the risk, and some promising broad-based approaches to prevention.

INCIDENCE OF CHILD FATALITIES

In 2003, the child fatality rate (ages 0–19) for the United States was 31.0/100,000 children while the infant mortality rate (ages 0–1) was 7.0/100,000 births (Hoyert, Mathews, Menacker, Strobino, & Guyer, 2006). For all causes and all children 0–19, there were 2,512 homicides with an incident rate of 3.1/100,000 (Hoyert et al., 2006). It was estimated that 2,000 children that year died from fatal child abuse. As will be mentioned later, this number is an estimate and likely underrepresents the true number of child abuse fatalities. Since data on child fatalities have always been estimates, knowing whether the incidence is rising or falling is hard to determine. Young children, however, account for a majority of these deaths. Children under 6 years old account for 86% of the deaths while infants under 1 year account for 46% of deaths.

The most common cause of child maltreatment deaths is abusive head trauma (AHT), which has a mortality rate of approximately 30/100,000 births (Keenan et al., 2003) in the first year of life. Given the discrepancy in the incidence of AHT deaths and the child fatality rate, it is important to understand the factors that lead to the determination of the cause of death in a child.

CAUSES OF CHILD FATALITIES

Although fatal abuse is most commonly thought of as the violent shaking or beating of a child who subsequently dies of the brain trauma, there are other etiologies:

- Suffocation—deliberate, coincident with cosleeping
- Munchausen Syndrome by Proxy (MSBP)
- Poisoning—deliberate or MSBP
- Severe malnutrition as a result of severe neglect or nonorganic failure to thrive

Assessment of each of these forms of child abuse fatalities has a variety of challenges. This chapter will focus on three of them: abusive head trauma, suffocation, and neglect. Death by poisoning as a result of MSBP is very uncommon and the overall management of children who are suspected of being victims of MSBP is too distinct a phenomenon, with different risk factors and complicated implications, to be part of this volume (see Rosenberg, 1987, and Rosenberg, 2003, for a review).

CHILD DEATH INVESTIGATION

To understand how to evaluate child fatalities from these three causes, it is important to first understand the status of cause of death determination in the United States. No uniform system for death determination exists in this country. There is a variety of coroner or medical examiner systems, which vary among the states and often even within each state (see Figure 4.1).

In general, medical examiners are forensic pathologists trained in autopsy and forensic investigations, while coroners are elected or appointed offi cials who may or may not be physicians. Currently, there are around 2,000 distinct jurisdictions for death investigation in the United States, ranging in size from a small county to an entire state. Unfortunately, there are only about 1,000 forensic pathologists in the United States, and even fewer with specialized training in pediatric pathology. The subsequent variability that exists in investigation technique and quality is one reason for a significant underestimate in the approximately 2,000 child abuse fatalities annually in the United States. In order to address this problem, a more uniform child fatality review process was developed (Covington, Foster, & Rich, 2005).

Ideal Process for Child Death Investigation

The ideal process for fatality assessment has two phases: the death investigation and the child fatality review. The death investigation of any sudden and unexpected death in a child has three stages: scene investigation, autopsy, and collateral history from involved professionals.

The scene investigation has been made popular recently by television crime shows such as *CSI*, but it is the stage of the investigation that is most likely overlooked or inadequately completed. Many jurisdictions will utilize specific protocols for infant or childhood scene investigation and use trained homicide detectives to respond to the home or location of death immediately after the child dies. In the ideal situation, trained police officers will respond

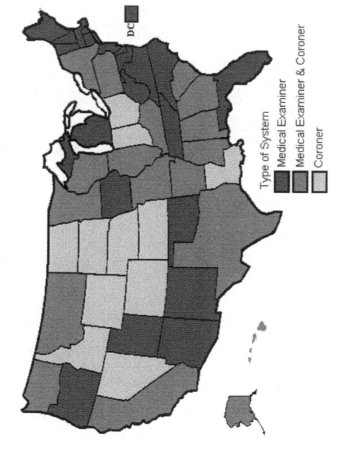

FIGURE 4.1 System of death investigation by state.
Figure courtesy of David Fowler, MB ChB, Chief Medical Examiner, State of Maryland.

immediately to the scene of every sudden and unexplained child death. They will conduct a thorough scene investigation, often in conjunction with investigators from the medical examiner's office. The scene investigation will assess where the child was found, who the child was with, and what the child was doing at the time of death. In the case of a child found dead in a bed or crib, the sleep position the child was placed in and the position the child was found in will be determined as well as the presence of other objects in the bed. Forensic collection of blood or other bodily fluids should be taken as well as pictures of the entire scene.

The autopsy of a dead child also must be done by a pathologist familiar with causes of childhood death. A complete autopsy will include an external examination, internal examination, histological examination, toxicological studies, microbiological tests, and metabolic screening for genetic conditions. Most infant deaths should include a skeletal survey to evaluate for occult or healing fractures and often crucial organs such as the brain, eyes, or heart need to be sent to pathological specialists for evaluation.

Finally, before determining a cause of death, the coroner or medical examiner should evaluate the past medical and social history of the child. The past medical history can help elucidate the cause of death in circumstances such as children with seizure disorders or cardiac conditions. A high-risk social situation may lead to an undetermined cause of death in a child whose evaluation fails to find a cause of death. The term SUDI (sudden unexplained death in infancy) is often used in this case. Unfortunately, there is not universal agreement on use of the term and it varies from locale to locale. In Maryland, for instance, this term is used to describe the cause of death in infants who died suddenly and unexpectedly, but do not meet the criteria for SIDS because of potential social or environmental risk factors. Over the past decade, the rate of SIDS has decreased significantly, but the SUDI rate has increased, likely because of the reclassification into the latter group of children who used to be called SIDS before thorough investigations were routine (American Academy of Pediatrics, 2005).

Because of the variation across jurisdictions, national groups have been working to standardize protocols for infant death investigation. Examples of these protocols for infant death scene investigation and autopsy can be found at:

http://www.childdeathreview.org/investigation.htm
http://www.cdc.gov/SIDS/PDF/SUIDIforms.pdf

Child Fatality Review

The second part of child death assessment is the child fatality review process. Child fatality review (CFR) began in the late 1970s in a few locations with local teams being founded in Los Angeles, Oregon, and North Carolina with the goal of better identifying child abuse fatalities (Michigan Public Health Institute, 2005a). In the 1990s, studies from Missouri (Ewigman, Kivlahan, & Land, 1993), New York (Herman-Giddens, 1999), and Colorado (Crume, DiGuiseppi, Byers, Sirotnak, & Garrett, 2002) demonstrated that fatalities due to child abuse were significantly underreported (up to 61%, more than doubling the reported rate), and the CFR process was able to better classify the deaths.

In 1993, the federal Child Abuse Prevention and Treatment Act (CAPTA) required states to include information on child death review in their program plans. In the past decade, CFR teams have been formed in all 50 states and the District of Columbia; many teams focus on determining the cause of all child deaths, not just those secondary to child abuse. Many teams will consist of medical, forensic, law enforcement, social services, school, and citizen representatives who meet regularly to review all sudden and unexpected child deaths.

The CFR process is best seen as a quality control/process improvement system. While there is some variation in focus among teams, the majority of teams are a multidisciplinary group that conducts reviews of all unexpected childhood deaths in a community with the purpose of better understanding why the child died in order to prevent future deaths. This goal is broader than the original teams, which only sought to identify fatal child abuse, but the broader goal has helped create process improvements in the identification of fatal child abuse.

One of the primary objectives of CFR teams is to "ensure the accurate identification and uniform, consistent reporting of the cause and manner of every child death" (Michigan Public Health Institute, 2005b). By reviewing each death in a locale, each community can ensure that their death investigators are conducting appropriate scene investigations and autopsies, which are crucial in cause of death determination. Other objectives of child death review include improving agency responses to evaluating deaths in general and homicides in particular, and protecting other siblings in a family (Michigan Public Health Institute, 2005b). Each of these efforts in a community will lead to improved case ascertainment as well as prevention of future deaths from fatal child abuse.

For more information on local and state CFR teams, a "how-to" manual, and further information, visit the National Matermal Child Care (MCH) Center for Child Death Review's Web site at http://www.childdeathreview.org.

CHILD ABUSE FATALITY TYPOLOGIES

Abusive Head Trauma (AHT)

AHT is the leading cause of fatal child abuse cases in infants and is one of the leading causes of death in infants under the age of 1 year. Many cases are very clear-cut, as when a child is found with bruising, multiple fractures, head bleeds, retinal hemorrhages, and other signs of trauma. However, when a child is found dead and has only a subdural hematoma and retinal hemorrhages, the certainty of the cause of death being child abuse is less clear. There are other conditions that can have this presentation such as glutaric aciduria type I, unintentional trauma to a child with an enlarged subarchnoid space (which may increase the fragility of the bridging veins making them susceptible to rupture with less force), and other conditions.

A complete review of the literature and controversies surrounding diagnosis of fatal AHT is not feasible here, but other references are included in Table 4.1 later in this chapter. For anyone other than forensic pathologists involved in cases of suspected child abuse fatalities, the major points to remember are:

1. Obtain a complete history of the last 24–48 hours of the child's life including the eating and sleeping pattern.
2. Obtain a complete social and family history.
3. Contact a local or regional child abuse consultant (available from the nearest children's hospital, school of medicine department of pediatrics, or the American Academy of pediatrics (AAP) Section on Child Abuse and Neglect).

Suffocation Versus SIDS

Sudden Infant Death Syndrome (SIDS) was first defined in the 1970s by consensus statement. SIDS is a diagnosis of exclusion, defined as a child dying under the age of 1 year with no known cause. The vast majority of children who die from SIDS are under 6 months and found in an unsafe sleep position, such as prone sleeping. The confusion and debate among professionals between SIDS and suffocation has been going on from the first SIDS description. The first hypothesis for etiology of SIDS, the apnea hypothesis (infants get recurrent episodes of apnea, then later die of SIDS), was based primarily on the deaths of infants whose mothers were repeatedly suffocating them (Firstman & Talan, 1997; Steinschneider; 1972). Suffocating an infant with a pillow can leave no findings on autopsy and a completely negative scene investigation.

Guidelines for the distinction of the two conditions are now available (AAP, Hymel, Committee on Child Abuse and Neglect, & National Association of Medical Examiners, 2006) and rely on following the best practices of scene investigation and autopsy. There are no data to suggest that SIDS is genetically determined. Therefore, families in which two or more children have died and have been called "SIDS cases" should absolutely have a complete investigation and be under heightened suspicion for either suffocation or a genetic abnormality.

Neglect

Over half of child abuse fatalities are due to neglect. Once again, the obvious cases of children being locked in rooms who starve to death are not a challenge to investigators. What is often challenging is determining whether civil or criminal neglect has occurred in a given case (such as an unsupervised 10-month-old falling from an apartment window with a torn screen). The continuum of supervision lapses leads to different responses. On one end is the prosecution of parents for leaving children alone with access to firearms. On the other is the acceptance that a child who dies in a motor vehicle crash who was not in an appropriate car seat is still an awful "accident." With regard to supervision, the American Academy of Pediatrics believes that supervisory neglect occurs whenever a caregiver's supervisory decisions or behaviors place a child in his or her care at significant (and often ongoing) risk for physical, emotional, or psychological harm (American Academy of Pediatrics, Hymel, & Committee on Child Abuse and Neglect, 2006).

RISK FACTORS FOR FATAL CHILD ABUSE

Many of the risk factors for physical child abuse overlap with those for child abuse fatalities, as previous child maltreatment is a strong risk factor for child homicide (Sabotta & Davis, 1992; Sorenson & Peterson, 1994). Older retrospective studies have found both maternal and child risk factors for fatal child abuse, as highlighted in Table 4.1.

More recent work has taken advantage of statewide assessment systems. Better characterization of perpetrator and household characteristics has emerged (and it overlaps with risk factors for AHT). Children in households with unrelated parents have been shown to have an eightfold increase in risk of death as compared to those with two biological parents and children with step, foster, or adoptive parents had a fourfold increase in risk compared to those with relatives in the home (Stiffman, Schnitzer, Adam, Kruse, & Ewigman, 2002).

Over an 8-year study period using Missouri's child fatality data, in 2005, Schnitzer and Ewigman found that children who lived with unrelated adults had a 50-fold increase in risk of death over children who lived with two parents. This study as well as other studies describing perpetrator characteristics of children who die from AHT (Keenan et al., 2003; Starling & Holden, 2000), have found that males are the perpetrators in approximately 70% of deaths, with the child's father followed by a nonbiologic male as the most common perpetrators.

TABLE 4.1   Risk Factors for Fatal Child Abuse

Maternal Risk Factors	Studies
Young maternal age	Brenner et al.,1999; Cummings, Theis, & Rivara, 1994; Keenan et al., 2003; Overpeck et al., 1998; Scholer, Mitchel, & Ray, 1997; Seigel et al., 1996; Winpisinger et al., 1991
Less than HS education	Brenner et al., 1999; Overpeck, et al., 1998; Scholer, Mitchel, & Ray, 1997; Winpisinger et al.,1991
Late or no prenatal care	Brenner et al., 1999; Cummings, Theis, & Rivara, 1994; Overpeck et al., 1998; Scholer, Mitchel, & Ray, 1997; Seigel et al., 1996; Winpisinger et al., 1991
Unmarried parents	Brenner et al., 1999; Keenan et al., 2003; Overpeck et al., 1998; Scholer, Mitchel, & Ray, 1997; Starling & Holden, 2000; Winpisinger et al., 1991
Black race	Brenner et al., 1999; Cummings, Theis, & Rivara, 1994; Keenan et al., 2003; Overpeck et al., 1998; Seigel et al., 1996
Child Risk Factors	
Male gender	Cummings, Theis, & Rivara, 1994; Keenan et al., 2003; Scholer, Mitchel, & Ray, 1997
Low birth weight	Brenner et al., 1999; Emerick, Foster, & Campbell, 1986; Seigel et al., 1996; Winpisinger et al., 1991
Multiple birth	Keenan et al., 2003
Previously documented maltreatment	Sabotta & Davis, 1992; Sorenson & Peterson, 1994

PREVENTION

Utilization of risk factors has led to a variety of primary preventive strategies targeted at high-risk populations. There are two general prevention strategies: parent education and home visitation. Approaches to parent education (e.g., Parents As Teachers [PAT] and Healthy Families America) hope that giving new parents increased knowledge about parenting and child development will reduce the likelihood that a child will be abused in that family (for a review of parent education programs see the David and Lucille Packard Foundation *Future of Children* report, 1999). These programs are not specific for child fatality prevention and have mixed success in preventing nonfatal child abuse.

Thirty-five years ago, Gray, Cutler, Dean, and Kempe (1979) showed that it was possible to identify children at risk of physical abuse and neglect by observing the parents' interaction with their infants prenatally and perinatally. The provision of a lay home visitor to these families reduced the level and severity of physical abuse and neglect. These were not controlled studies, but indicated that giving stressed, at-risk parents someone to contact could potentially prevent abusive and neglectful situations. While not specifically shown to reduce childhood mortality, Olds's home visiting studies using public health nurses intervening with high-risk mothers pre- and postnatally have shown significant reductions in rates of child abuse reports, subsequent alcohol abuse, criminal behavior, and other childhood negative well-being outcomes (Olds et al., 1997)

More recent primary preventive strategies that show promise focus on newborn parent education about AHT. A recently published effective strategy goes beyond just warning parents to "never shake a baby," and includes giving all parents of newborns a pamphlet about AHT and crying, showing parents a video, and having them sign a "commitment statement" to warn any caregiver about the dangers of shaking babies (Dias et al., 2005). This relatively simple nursery intervention reduced the incidence of AHT in western New York by 61%.

The CFR process itself may lead to a reduction in child deaths. Works from Georgia (Luallen et al., 1998) and Arizona (Rimsza, Schackner, Bowen, & Marshall, 2002) have shown a reduction in unintentional deaths. While a decrease has not shown the same potential in abusive fatalities, the same process of identifying and modifying risk factors may help. Alternatively, proper review and having well-functioning death investigation processes may actually initially increase the incidence due to improved classification.

Unfortunately, there is no single effective strategy to modify risk factors and prevent fatal child abuse deaths. One of the challenges is that given the low overall incidence of childhood abuse fatalities, coupled with the high prevalence of these risk factors, predictive value of any or a combination of factors will always end up low. Any intervention needs to reach a large number of individuals in order to prevent one death. It is likely that a variety of approaches are needed to prevent child fatalities. Including education in the newborn period, new parent support via home visitation, and community involvement in assuring healthy families will be the only way to significantly reduce the rates of fatal child abuse.

REFERENCES

American Academy of Pediatrics, Task Force on Sudden Infant Death Syndrome. (2005). The changing concept of sudden infant death syndrome: Diagnostic coding shifts, controversies regarding the sleeping environment, and new variables to consider in reducing risk. *Pediatrics, 116,* 1245–1255.

American Academy of Pediatrics, Hymel, K. P., Committee on Child Abuse and Neglect, & National Association of Medical Examiners. (2006). Distinguishing sudden infant death syndrome from child abuse fatalities. *Pediatrics, 118,* 421–427.

American Academy of Pediatrics, Hymel, K. P., & Committee on Child Abuse and Neglect. (2006). When is lack of supervision neglect? *Pediatrics, 118,* 1296–1298.

Brenner, R. A., Overpeck, M. D., Trumble, A. C., DerSimonian, R., & Berendes, H. (1999). Deaths attributable to injuries in infants, United States, 1983–1991. *Pediatrics, 103,* 968–974.

Covington, C. M., Foster, V., & Rich, S. K. (2005). *The child death review case reporting system: Systems manual.* National MCH Center for Child Death Review. Retrieved September 24, 2006, from .http://www.childdeathreview.org/reports/CDR%20Systems%20Manual.pdf

Crume, T. L., DiGuiseppi, C., Byers, T., Sirotnak, A. P., & Garrett, C. J. (2002). Under ascertainment of Child Maltreatment Fatalities by Death Certificates, 1990–1998. *Pediatrics, 110,* e18.

Cummings, P., Theis, M. K. A., & Rivara, F. P. (1994). Infant injury death in Washington State, 1981 through 1990. *Archives of Pediatrics and Adolescent Medicine, 148,* 1021–1026.

David and Lucile Packard Foundation. (1999). Home visiting: Recent program evaluations. *The Future of Children: Vol. 9.*

Dias, M. S., Smith, K., deGuehery, K., Mazur, P., Li, V., & Shaffer, M. L. (2005). Preventing abusive head trauma among infants and young children: A hospital-based, parent education program. *Pediatrics, 115,* 470–477.

Emerick, S. J., Foster, L. R., & Campbell, D. T. (1986). Risk factors for traumatic infant death in Oregon, 1973 to 1982. *Pediatrics, 77,* 518–522.

Ewigman, B., Kivlahan, C., & Land, G. (1993). The Missouri child fatality study: Underreporting of maltreatment fatalities among children younger than five years of age, 1983 through 1986. *Pediatrics, 91,* 330–337.

Firstman, R., & Talan, J. (1997). *The death of innocents.* New York: Bantam Books.

Gray, J. D., Cutler, C. A., Dean, J. G., & Kempe, C. H. (1979). Prediction and prevention of child abuse and neglect. *Journal of Social Issues, 35,* 127–139.

Herman-Giddens, M. E. (1999). Underascertainment of child abuse mortality in the United States. *Journal of the American Medical Association, 282,* 463–467.

Hoyert, D. L., Mathews, T. J., Menacker, F., Strobino, D. M., & Guyer, B. (2006). Annual summary of vital statistics: 2004. *Pediatrics, 117,*168–183.

Keenan, H. T., Runyan, D. K., Marshall, S. W., Nocera, M. A., Merten, D. F., & Sinal, S. H. (2003). A population-based study of inflicted traumatic brain injury in young children. *Journal of the American Medical Association, 290,* 621–626.

Luallen, J. J., Rochat, R. W., Smith, S. M., O'Neil, J., Rogers, M. Y., & Bolen, J. C. (1998). Child fatality review in Georgia: A young system demonstrates its potential for identifying preventable deaths. *Southern Medical Journal, 91,* 414–419.

Michigan Public Health Institute. (2005a). *History of child death review in the United States.* Retrieved October 2, 2006, from http://www.childdeathreview.org/Promo/history.pdf

Michigan Public Health Institute. (2005b). *The child death review process.* Retrieved October 2, 2006, from http://www.childdeathreview.org/cdrprocess.htm

Olds, D. L., Eckenrode, J., Henderson, C. R., Kitzman, H., Powers, J., Cole, R., et al. (1997). Long-term effects of home visitation on maternal life course and child abuse and neglect. Fifteen-year follow-up of a randomized trial. *Journal of the American Medical Association, 27,* 278, 637–643.

Overpeck, M. D., Brenner, R. A., Trumble, A. C., Trifiletti, L. B., & Berendes, H. W. (1998). Risk factors for infant homicide in the United States. *New England Journal of Medicine, 339,* 1211–1216.

Rimsza, M. E., Schackner, R. A., Bowen, K. A., & Marshall, W. (2002). Can child deaths be prevented? The Arizona Child Fatality Review Program experience. *Pediatrics, 110,* e11.

Roche, J. A., Fortin, G., Labbe, J., Brown, J., & Chadwick, D. (2005). The work of Ambroise Tardieu: The first definitive description of child abuse. *Child Abuse & Neglect, 29,* 325–334.

Rosenberg, D. A. (1987).Web of deceit: a literature review of Munchausen Syndrome by Proxy. *Child Abuse & Neglect: The International Journal, 11,* 547–563.

Rosenberg, D. A. (2003). Munchausen Syndrome by Proxy: medical diagnostic criteria. *Child Abuse & Neglect: The International Journal, 27,* 421–430.

Sabotta, E. E., & Davis, R. L. (1992). Fatality after report to a child abuse registry in Washington State, 1973–1986. *Child Abuse & Neglect: The International Journal, 16,* 627–635.

Schnitzer, P. G., & Ewigman, B. G. (2005). Child deaths resulting from inflicted injuries: Household risk factors and perpetrator characteristics. *Pediatrics, 116,* 687–693.

Scholer, S. J., Mitchel, E. F., & Ray, W. A. (1997). Predictors of injury mortality in early childhood. *Pediatrics, 100,* 342–347.

Siegel, C. D., Graves, P., Maloney, K., Norris, J. M., Calonge, B. N., & Lezotte, D. (1996). Mortality from intentional and unintentional injury among infants of young mothers in Colorado, 1986 to 1992. *Archives of Pediatrics & Adolescent Medicine, 150,* 1077–1083.

Sorenson, S. B., & Peterson, J. G. (1994). Traumatic child death and documented maltreatment history, Los Angeles. *American Journal of Public Health, 84,* 623–627.

Starling, S. P., & Holden, J. R. (2000). Perpetrators of abusive head trauma: A comparison of two geographic populations. *Southern Medical Journal, 93,* 463–465.

Steinschneider, A. (1972). Prolonged apnea and the sudden infant death syndrome: Clinical and laboratory observations. *Pediatrics, 50,* 646–654.

Stiffman, M. N., Schnitzer, P. G., Adam, P., Kruse, R. L., & Ewigman, B. G. (2002). Child deaths resulting from inflicted injuries: Household risk factors and perpetrator characteristics. *Pediatrics, 116,* 687–693.

U.S. Advisory Board on Child Abuse and Neglect. (1995). *A nation's shame: Fatal child abuse and neglect in the United States.* Fifth Report. Washington, DC: U.S. Department of Health and Human Services.

Winpisinger, K. A., Hopkins, R. S., Indian, R. W., & Hostetler, J. R. (1991). Risk factors for childhood homicides in Ohio: A birth certificate-based case-control study. *American Journal of Public Health, 81,* 1052–1054.

CHAPTER 5

Prediction of Homicide of and by Battered Women

Jacquelyn C. Campbell

Homicide is now the second leading cause of death (after unintentional injury) in the United States for African American women aged 15 to 34 (Centers for Disease Control and Prevention [CDC], 2000). It is the third leading cause of death in the same age group for young Native American women (after unintentional injuries and suicide). The rate of homicide per 100,000 for young African American women was 13.3 in the year 2000, as compared with 1.3 per 100,000 for females overall (Department of Health and Human Services [DHHS], 2000; Fox & Zawitz, 2004). This rate for African American females is exceeded only by that for African American males (84.9 per 100,000) and Latino males (33.5 per 100,000) in the same age group (15 to 34 years). The homicide rate for African American women of all ages is higher than that of men of all races (10.3 per 100,000 vs. 10 per 100,000), and approximately four times the rate for white women (DHHS, 2000). Overall, men are 3.4 times more likely than women to be murdered, but female intimates are currently about 4 times more likely to be killed than are male intimate partners (Fox & Zawitz, 2004). African American, Native American, and Alaskan Native women are also disproportionately at risk for intimate partner homicide.[1]

HOMICIDE AND BATTERING

Homicides involving women as victim or perpetrator have different dynamics from those more often studied, between two males (Mercy & Saltzman, 1989; Moracco, Runyan, & Butts, 1998). For example, 90% of women murdered are killed by men, men who are most often a family member, spouse, or ex-partner (Campbell, 1992; Fox & Zawitz, 2004). Approximately 40%–50% of murdered women are killed by a husband, lover, or estranged same when hand counts of homicide records are performed (Campbell, 1992; Campbell et al., 2003; Moracco et al., 1998). When homicide statistics are based on the Uniform Crime Reports data, there is no perpetrator category for ex-boyfriend or ex-girlfriend, a category that accounts for as much as 20% of the perpetrators of intimate partner homicide of women, or femicide (Campbell et al, 2003; Langford, Isaac, & Kabat, 1998). Therefore, the "official" estimate of 30%–40% of femicides being categorized as intimate partner homicide is a serious undercount.

Approximately two-thirds to three-quarters of murders of women by intimate partners or ex-partners are preceded by documented domestic violence against the female partner before they were killed (Campbell, 1981, 1992, Campbell et al., 2003; Moracco et al., 1998). Homicide of a female partner or ex-partner followed by suicide of the perpetrator is another form of homicide of women wherein a history of female partner abuse is the most usual pattern (Koziol-McLain et al., 2006; Morton, Runyan, Moracco, & Butts, 1998).

When women kill, they usually kill a family member. They most often kill husbands, ex-husbands, and lovers, and again there most often is a documented history of wife assault (approximately 75% of cases) (Campbell, 1992; Moracco et al., 1998). In addition, women are far more likely than men to kill during an incident of domestic violence when they are being attacked by an intimate partner. Women usually kill when the male victim was the first to commit a violent act (strike a blow, show a weapon), commonly termed *victim precipitation* in homicide research (Campbell, 1992; Daly & Wilson, 1988; Jurik & Winn, 1990; Mann, 1990).

NEED FOR PREVENTION

From these data it is clear that one of the major ways to decrease spousal homicide is to identify and intervene with abused women at risk to be killed by or to kill their abuser. Research has demonstrated that the majority of battered women eventually leave their abusers (Campbell, Miller, Cardwell, & Belknap,

1994; Campbell, O'Sullivan, Roehl, & Webster, 2005). The trajectory of serious intimate partner violence (IPV), however, is often an increase in severity and frequency over time (Johnson, 2006; Straus & Gelles, 1990) that may culminate in a homicide unless the woman leaves or the man receives either evidence-based intervention to reduce IPV or is held accountable through the criminal justice system. In addition, women are often highly at risk for homicide and repeat severe violence for the first year after they have left their abusers (with the first three months especially dangerous) or when it is clear to the abuser that the woman is leaving for good (Campbell et al., 2003; Campbell et al., 2005; Daly & Wilson, 1988; Hart, 1988; Moracco et al., 1998).

From in-depth interviews with battered women, it is apparent that the majority carefully weigh the pluses and minuses of the overall relationship, both in terms of their safety and well-being and that of their children (Campbell et al., 1994; Campbell, Rose, Kub, & Nedd, 1998). Many, however, have not realistically appraised the potential for homicide. Even though the majority of women interviewed had at least considered the possibility of homicide, they might have found it too frightening to dwell on or may underestimate their risk.

The possibility of reading in the paper that an abused woman seen in a research or safety planning or clinical interaction has been killed is a constant concern to advocates and professionals. Advocates in wife abuse shelters are extremely concerned about women leaving the shelter without knowing how dangerous their situations might be. Thus clinicians who work with abused women need to make sure women realize the potential of homicide in their situation and to give them a way to realistically assess their risk of homicide. This is both an ethical and a legal imperative, as well as an aid to sleeping well at night (Campbell, 2005; Hart, 1988).

For health care professionals, there is some similarity to explaining the risks of cancer to smokers so that they can make their own decisions about actions to be taken. Some analogies also can be made to the appraisal done for risk of suicide by physical and mental health care professionals wherein a clinical assessment is done, and if the risk is considered great, action is taken to ensure the person's safety. This type of unilateral professional action might come into play for an abused woman when her emotional trauma is so great that the professional believes she is unable to make reasonable decisions about her own safety. Yet the clinicians' "duty to warn" battered women about their risk of homicide, even though primarily a clinical issue, can be better informed by statistical prediction of dangerousness than by purely clinical estimations by themselves (Pinard & Pagani, 2001).

The background on homicide of or by abused women presented above establishes the need for assessment of risk of IP homicide. This chapter also includes discussion of issues related to clinical prediction as contrasted with formal legal prediction and a description of the danger signs lists, risk assessment instruments, or systems of lethality assessment danger that have been published. The degree to which they have been subjected to psychometric testing will be presented. The chapter concludes with a presentation of the Danger Assessment (DA) instrument for assessing risk of homicide in battering relationships, along with recent validity data (Campbell et al., 2005; Campbell, Webster, & Glass, in press).

PREDICTION ISSUES

Clinical prediction of dangerousness in situations of battering has legal implications. A series of court decisions during the past 20 years has held clinicians negligent for not adequately predicting dangerousness and subsequently for not at least protecting clients as potential victims, and in some states for not providing warnings to potential victims of clients (Hart, 1988). General agreement by legal experts is that if a therapist decides that her or his patient is a serious danger to someone else, the therapist must warn potential victims (Small, 1985).

This legal mandate is especially pertinent where therapists are conducting couple counseling or intervention groups for batterers, because of the demonstrated risk of homicide in battering relationships. It places the onus of responsibility on the therapist for assessing for potential for homicide, as well as for warning potential victims. Therefore, all couple counseling needs to include assessment for abuse done with each partner separately and, where abuse is found, assessment for homicide potential.

Homicide potential also needs to be assessed in cases where men are in batterer intervention programs whether or not they still are living with their partners, and means of partner notification and appropriate safety planning with partners established. Ex-spouses are known to be potentially lethal to their formerly abused female partners (Campbell, 1992; Campbell et al., 2003). In all cases where the clinician judges homicide potential to be high, both the abused partner and the police and/or probation officer need to be notified. In cases of high potential for homicide, the law is clear that the duty to warn takes precedence over confidentiality. There has also been at least one case where a probation department has been successfully sued for failing to adequately supervise a case with well-known intimate partner homicide risk factors, and the probationer killed his partner (Lilienthal, 2004).

Although there are no cases that have been adjudicated for legal precedent, analogous cases have been settled out of court involving the health care system. Research has established that abused women later killed have been seen in the health care system (Sharps, Koziol-McLain, et al., 2001; Wadman & Muelleman, 1999) and it has been clearly established practice that victims of domestic violence be assessed and appropriately referred by health care professionals since 1996 (Joint Commission on the Accreditation of Healthcare Organizations [JCAHO], 2006).

Clinical Judgment of Risk Assessment

To determine the degree of homicide risk, clinicians often make use of intuitive or clinical judgment prediction based on the clinician's training, experience, and expertise (see Chapter 2). This intuitive judgment also involves the implicit assumptions and biases of the clinician (Miller & Morris, 1988) and is consistently judged as slightly but significantly less accurate than statistical prediction in the prediction of violence (Ægisdóttir, et al., 2006; Hilton, Harris, & Rice, 2006).

Psychological testing (such as using a psychopathy evaluation instrument) that has been used in the patient's clinical assessment may improve the accuracy of clinical prediction. Clinical judgment also may be based on reading of literature or workshops that the clinician has attended on intimate partner violence as well as experience in the field. Some of that material contains lists of danger signals to watch for, signs that have been developed from a mixture of research results from retrospective studies (examining the characteristics of homicide cases after they have occurred) and clinical experience of the author or trainer. These lists can help prediction accuracy in terms of helping clinicians remember what factors to consider but have not been subjected to prospective testing (research that tries to predict actual or near lethality from the factors identified).

Statistically based prediction using psychometrically developed and tested (or actuarial) instruments is not completely accurate either, especially in the instruments' present state of development in the area of spousal homicide. However, based on meta-analyses of other violence instruments, such instruments are more accurate than clinical judgments by themselves (Hilton et al., 2006). At the present time, the best assessment is probably a combination of a psychometrically tested instrument or system, the assessment of the victim of domestic violence, and an experienced clinician's judgment (Campbell, 2005; Pinard & Pagani, 2001).

The criminal justice system may use experts' predictions of homicide in battering situations in decisions about incarceration, probation, and/or court-mandated batterer intervention. This use may be formal, as in court testimony, or informal, as in communication between a probation officer and the clinicians treating the batterer in the case. The formal use of prediction for arrest and sentencing decisions demands as great a degree of accuracy as possible.

Risk Assessment Instruments

As the field of risk assessment in domestic violence cases has developed, instruments and systems with cutoff scores or levels of risk have been developed with various amounts of research conducted on their use. Clinical advice given on matters of life and death probably would involve drastic measures by the client, and the clinician must be sure of the accuracy of any cutoff score. Only predictive validity testing, studies that determine the accuracy of the instrument in predicting actual homicide, gives a cutoff score that provides the kind of support necessary either to give clients definitive advice about avoiding a homicide or to advise the courts or other agencies on the statistical probability of an abusive or abused partner committing homicide.

Most of the instruments with cutoff scores or levels of risk in the domestic violence field are designed to determine the level of risk of re-assault or recurrence of IPV. These are described in detail in Chapter 4 in this volume. Although the risk of homicide and risk of re-assault in domestic violence cases involve the same risk factors for the most part, they are not exactly the same, and the weight they should be given in prediction of homicide versus re-assault may be different.

For instance, substance abuse on the part of the abuser is a significant risk factor for re-assault but not nearly as strong for IP homicide of women (Sharps et al., 2001). Also important are the protective actions that IPV victims take and the protectiveness of the system where the couple resides. For instance, in a city where violation of an order of protection brings swift and sure criminal justice response, a dangerous batterer may be prevented from committing a homicide. Prior arrest for domestic violence may be an important predictor of IP homicide. If an abused woman finds protection by going to a wife abuse shelter, her actions may mitigate the potential for homicide (Campbell et al., 2005). This overlap is illustrated in Figure 5.1.

Prediction of homicide rather than re-assault is especially difficult because homicide is rarer than other forms of violence. Spousal homicide is even rarer and therefore even more difficult to predict. Because battering

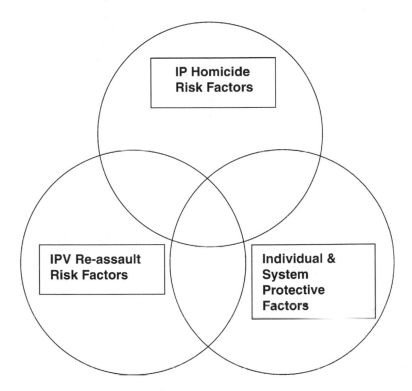

FIGURE 5.1 Overlap in risk factors.

is the most frequent relationship precursor of spousal homicide, it makes sense to design a predictive instrument around characteristics related to abuse. Yet this design makes the number of occurrences, homicides in abusive relationships, even smaller. To assess for homicide potential and follow abusive couples (somewhere around 3–4 million per year) over time to see which few end up as homicide cases (around 1,600 per year) to definitively establish predictive validity would involve huge sample sizes, be enormously expensive and time consuming, and be unethical if interventions were not implemented.

If the national homicide files were used to identify the homicides, any such effort would be hampered by the inaccuracies of national homicide files, especially in terms of relationship category (exclusion of ex-boyfriend/girlfriend perpetrators) (Campbell, 1992; Wilson, 1991). The picture is confounded further because whether or not a serious assault becomes a homicide may be determined by the speed and/or quality of emergency response rather than by the relationship, perpetrator, and victim characteristics that can be measured and used for prediction. Finally, careful prediction validity assessment would be necessary to determine how various risk factors should be weighted. Common sense dictates that certain factors would be more predictive of homicide than others. Yet without a statistical evaluation, designation of which risk factors should be taken more seriously than others is also premature.

Published Lists of Danger Signs

In the prior version of this text (Campbell, 1995), lists of lethality risk signs by Sonkin, Martin, and Walker (1985), Barbara Hart (1988), and Murray Straus (1991), were described in detail. Although versions of all of these lists still are published in various texts and training materials, none have been subjected to prospective testing for predictive validity and therefore will not be further described here.

Those prediction risk factor lists concentrated on risk factors for male batterers killing their female partners. Although it happens slightly less often, abused women also kill their partners. Only studies by Browne (1987), Campbell (1992), and Moracco, Runyan, and Butts (1998) have concentrated on or included cases of battered women killing their abusers. The resulting risk factors from those studies were primarily related to the dangerousness of the male partner and therefore were almost the same as those predicting homicide of female partners. The one risk factor that was specific to abused women as potential perpetrators was her threats of suicide, but this has not yet been substantiated in subsequent predictive validity research with independent samples.

Danger Assessment Instrument

The Danger Assessment (DA) instrument, presented in Figure 5.2, is a form of statistical prediction, as contrasted with clinical prediction, because it is based on prior research (homicide record reviews) and has been validated in a case control study of homicide as well as tested for predictive accuracy of IPV re-assault (see Chapter 4). It was designed to be used in clinical settings as the basis of discussion with battered women by advocates in shelters, as well as by advocates in criminal and civil justice settings, health care professionals in emergency rooms and primary care settings, and social workers and psychologists in counseling situations.

DANGER ASSESSMENT

Jacquelyn C. Campbell, PhD, RN

Copyright 2004 Johns Hopkins University, School of Nursing
www.dangerassessment.org

Several risk factors have been associated with increased risk of homicides (murders) of women and men in violent relationships. We cannot predict what will happen in your case, but we would like you to be aware of the danger of homicide in situations of abuse and for you to see how many of the risk factors apply to your situation.

Using the calendar, please mark the approximate dates during the past year when you were abused by your partner or ex partner. Write on that date how bad the incident was according to the following scale:

1. Slapping, pushing; no injuries and/or lasting pain
2. Punching, kicking; bruises, cuts, and/or continuing pain
3. "Beating up"; severe contusions, burns, broken bones, miscarriage
4. Threat to use weapon; head injury, internal injury, permanent injury, miscarriage
5. Use of weapon; wounds from weapon

(If **any** of the descriptions for the higher number apply, use the higher number.)

Mark **Yes** or **No** for each of the following.
("He" refers to your husband, partner, ex-husband, ex-partner, or whoever is currently physically hurting you.)

Yes	No		
____	____	1.	Has the physical violence increased in severity or frequency over the past year?
____	____	2.	Does he own a gun?
		3.	Have you left him after living together during the past year?
			3a. (If have *never* lived with him, check here___)
____	____	4.	Is he unemployed?
		5.	Has he ever used a weapon against you or threatened you with a lethal weapon?
____	____		5a. (If yes, was the weapon a gun?____)
____	____	6.	Does he threaten to kill you?
____	____	7.	Has he avoided being arrested for domestic violence?
____	____	8.	Do you have a child that is not his?
____	____	9.	Has he ever forced you to have sex when you did not wish to do so?
____	____	10.	Does he ever try to choke you?
		11.	Does he use illegal drugs? By drugs, I mean "uppers" or amphetamines, speed, angel dust, cocaine, "crack", street drugs or mixtures.
____	____	12.	Is he an alcoholic or problem drinker?
		13.	Does he control most or all of your daily activities? (For instance: does he tell you who you can be friends with, when you can see your family, how much money you can use, or when you can take the car?
____	____		(If he tries, but you do not let him, check here: ____)
		14.	Is he violently and constantly jealous of you?
____	____		(For instance, does he say "If I can't have you, no one can.")
		15.	Have you ever been beaten by him while you were pregnant?
____	____		(If you have never been pregnant by him, check here: ____)
____	____	16.	Has he ever threatened or tried to commit suicide?
____	____	17.	Does he threaten to harm your children?
____	____	18.	Do you believe he is capable of killing you?
		19.	Does he follow or spy on you, leave threatening notes or messages on answering machine, destroy your property, or call you when you don't want him to?
____	____	20.	Have you ever threatened or tried to commit suicide?

_____ Total "Yes" Answers

**Thank you. Please talk to your nurse, advocate or counselor about
what the Danger Assessment means in terms of your situation.**

FIGURE 5.2 The Danger Assessment.

The DA could also be used by batterer intervention programs for lethality assessment and safety planning with partners as well as for informal prediction discussions with probation officers or other officers of the court responsible for presentencing investigations, recommendations about bail, and levels of supervision for probation for abusing men. With the new weighting of items and determination of levels of risk, it can also be used as evidence for formal prediction as in court sentencing situations.

Development and Psychometric Evaluation of the Danger Assessment

Table 5.1 is a summary of the developmental research for the Danger Assessment. The initial items on the instrument were developed from four retrospective research studies establishing risk factors in cases where battered women were killed or seriously injured by their abusers or where battered women killed or seriously injured their abusers (Berk, Berk, Loseke, & Rauma, 1983; Browne, 1987; Campbell, 1981, 1992; Fagan, Stewart, & Hansen, 1983).

The initial instrument development study (Study 1, Campbell, 1986) was conducted with a volunteer sample of 79 abused women from the community in two geographically and demographically distinct cities. The wording of all items has been clinically tested in shelter settings to be sure it is easily understandable by and in terminology common to abused women. All samples have included a substantial proportion of women of color and have been from a variety of settings (Table 5.1).

TABLE 5.1 Danger Assessment Studies

	1	2	3	4	5
N	79 abused	30 abused	52 abused	156 mixed	164 relationship
Setting	80% community	Shelter	36% ER 64% inpatient	Prenatal	Problem
	20% shelter		OB/GYN		
Ethnicity	46% minority	33% minority	62% minority	Black = 71 White = 46 Hispanic = 39	Black = 126 Nonblack = 37
Reliability	Alpha = .71	Test-retest = .94	Test-retest = .89	Alpha = .86	Alpha = .66
Validity	Construct (r)	Alpha = .60 Construct (r)	Alpha = .67 None	Construct (r)	Total sample (r)
	CTS = .55	Injury = .48		ISA = .75	ISA-P = .66
	Injury = .50 Tactic = .43			CTS = .49	ISA-NP = .44
Mean score	6.3	8.7	9.2 ER	.3 not abused	5.5
			8.3 inpatient	3.5 abused	

Where sufficient sample sizes have permitted, separate evaluations have been conducted by ethnic group. For instance, Study 4 in Table 5.1 was a Centers for Disease Control and Prevention funded prospective study of abuse during pregnancy (McFarlane, Parker, Soeken, & Bullock, 1992). The sample was approximately evenly divided into European American, African American, and Latino (mainly Mexican American). Concurrent validity was supported in all three groups, with the Latina women reporting lower scores on all measures of abuse, including the DA. The RAVE study concurrent validity evaluation of the DA was also equal in the same three major ethnic groups (Campbell et al., 2005).

Part of both the shelter and hospital studies (2 and 3 in Table 5.1) was an open-ended interview section asking women their perception of danger of being killed by their partners (Stuart & Campbell, 1989). Women then were asked what made them believe they were in danger or not. The majority of women perceiving a great amount of danger in both studies mentioned choking as a tactic used against them, which made them believe their partner might kill them. This item was added to the scale and in subsequent evaluations either did not affect or improved concurrent validity evaluations. Subsequent independent research has established the importance of attempted strangulation or "choking" as a potentially lethal act often used in dangerous abusive relationships (McClane, Strack, & Hawley, 2001).

Another item was added to the scale from the in-depth interview portion of the shelter study (2) that asked about the male partner's history of suicide threats and/or attempts. This item is related also to prior research on murder of abused women followed by suicide of the perpetrator (Morton et al., 1998) and also has been added. Addition of that item slightly improved both the reliability and validity estimates in the developmental studies. Both items were supported in the subsequent case control validity study (Campbell et al., in press; Koziol-McLain et al., 2006).

Calendar Evaluation of Pattern of Abuse

The pattern of abuse including severity and frequency is gauged on the Danger Assessment by presenting the woman with a calendar of the past year. The woman is asked to mark the approximate days when physically abusive incidents occurred, to estimate the amount of time the incident lasted, and to rank the incident on the scale presented on the Danger Assessment (Figure 5.2). If she indicates the incidents occur weekly or more often, only 3 months of the calendar need to be filled out. Most women have no problem filling out the calendar; they remember these incidents very well.

In the original scale development, women were asked the first question about increase in severity and frequency, then were asked to fill out the calendar, and then were asked the question again on the basis of the calendar. Some 38% of the women who initially said there was no increase answered the question yes after filling out the calendar, thereby indicating that the calendar portion is an important part of the instrument despite its adding 8 to 10 minutes to the 6- to 8-minute risk factor list administration time. In the two studies in which the calendar was not done (2 and 3), the increase of severity and/or frequency items substantially lowered internal consistency, also suggesting the efficacy of the calendar (Stuart & Campbell, 1989).

Judging from women's remarks as they complete the calendar, it seems to function as a consciousness-raising exercise, helping to cut through the denial and minimization that is a normal response to abuse (Campbell et al., 1998). These clinical observations are supported by the findings in the case control homicide study where only about half of abused women subsequently killed or almost killed accurately assessed their risk of lethality (Campbell, 2004; Campbell et al., 2003).

Thus, using women's general recall of whether or not the abuse is increasing in severity and/or frequency as a predictor of homicide may not be entirely accurate without some sort of specific cuing such as using the calendar.

Reliability

There is controversy about whether internal consistency reliability is an appropriate psychometric technique to use with risk assessment instruments wherein each item is considered to be an independent risk factor. With no consensus in the literature on this issue, alpha coefficient internal consistency estimations on the instrument were calculated (but they tend to be low). In the original study the alpha was .71. In subsequent studies it has ranged from .66 in a very small sample to .86 (see Table 5.1). In the two studies in which temporal stability (test-retest reliability) was assessed, it ranged from .89 to .94.

Convergent Validity

Convergent construct validity (positive relationships with similar constructs) of the DA was supported in the studies in Table 5.1 by correlations in the moderately strong range, with instruments measuring severity and/or frequency of abuse, the Conflict Tactics Scale (Straus & Gelles, 1990), the Index of Spouse Abuse (Hudson & McIntosh, 1981), and a rating of severity of worst injury incurred as a result of the abuse.

Validity in terms of the instrument successfully differentiating groups (concurrent predictive validity) also has been supported by the different means in the seven groups of abused women as seen in Table 5.1. These accurately reflect the differing degrees of severity of abuse one would expect in the different populations. The lowest scores were in the nonabused sample, with the next lowest in the prenatal sample, a group not known to be abused and expected to be early in an abuse pattern because of their relative youth and perhaps being protected from the worst of the abuse because of their pregnancy. In fact, very few women in this group reported increasing severity and/or frequency of battering during the pregnancy (McFarlane et al., 1992).

The highest scores were in the hospital emergency room group, a sample identified because of serious abuse-related injury. The next highest scores were from women in shelters, who often come to a shelter because of fear of a fatal incident. The samples of abused women from the community (Studies 1 and 5) had scores in the intermediary range.

Case Control Study

A multicity case (311 actual and 183 attempted femicides) control (426 abused women in the same cities) study (Campbell et al., 2003) provided additional support for the validity of the DA. All but one of the 15 items on the original DA were significant predictors of intimate partner femicide. That one item was victim suicidality. Since the item was meant to predict homicide of the abuse perpetrator (not tested in the case control study), and suicide is also potentially fatal to women and should therefore be assessed, the item was retained on the revised DA.

Wording of two other items from the original DA were changed to reflect information gained from the study and from clinical use of the DA. The item about perpetrator violence toward the children was changed to, "Does he threaten to harm your children?" This item was more predictive than asking about reported child abuse and also avoids the mandatory reporting of child abuse engendered by a positive response to the original form of the question.

The gun item (originally "Is there a gun in the home?") was changed slightly to, "Does he own a gun?" so that cases where he has left the home with his gun or lives elsewhere but owns a gun will elicit a positive answer.

The first two items from the original DA on severity and frequency were combined into one, since the multivariate analysis showed that each of these variables were equally predictive. Five other items were added that were significant predictors in the multivariate analysis of the 11-city femicide study, including items on stepchildren (her biological child but not his), batterer unemployment, estrangement, prior arrest, and stalking. The resulting revised

DA is 20 items long and is being used extensively, especially in advocacy settings (see Figure 5.2). Further information on the weighted scoring is available at www.dangerassessment.com.

Further reliability and concurrent validity support was found in the 11-city case control femicide study. The results demonstrated acceptable reliability of the DA among femicide victims (r = .80), attempted femicide victims (r = .75) and abused women (r = .74). Discriminant group validity was supported by a significant (p = .004) difference between the unweighted mean scores of cases (femicide victims = 7.4) and controls (abused women from the same cities = 3.2). Most importantly, using weightings based on the multivariate risk factor analysis of the femicide cases (Campbell et. al., 2003) resulted in a very good Receiver Operator Characteristic (ROC) analysis with 86.6% of the actual and 91.6% of the attempted femicide cases below the curve.

Women's Perception of Risk

Abused women's own perception of risk has been evaluated in several studies and found to be relatively accurate in assessing risk of re-assault (e.g., Goodman, Dutton, & Bennett, 2000; Weisz, Tolman, & Saunders, 2000); however, when evaluated in conjunction with the original 15-item DA, the combination of the DA and victim's perception was more precise than victim's perception alone (Heckert & Gondolf, 2004; Weisz et al., 2000).

Using the modified DA with weighted scoring, victim's perception of risk was almost as accurate (ROC = .60) as the DA (ROC = .64) in the RAVE study using re-assault as the outcome (Campbell, O'Sullivan, Roehl, & Webster, 2007). Women's perception of risk has not been evaluated in homicide studies except in the Campbell et al. (2003) case control femicide study, which found that less than half (46%) of women killed by their partners assessed their partner as capable of killing her according to family members prior to the homicide. Thus, abused women's perception of risk is not sufficient to accurately determine risk of homicide, although it is one important factor. The revised DA has a separate question asking about women's perception of risk of homicide.

FUTURE DIRECTIONS IN LETHALITY RISK ASSESSMENT

The Danger Assessment now has a substantive data base to support its use in domestic violence lethality assessment, but only for cases where a female is the victim of the abuse and the potential victim of homicide. Accuracy of the DA in predicting homicide risk in cases of homicide of male partners is as yet unknown. So far, most of the testing of the DA has been done by the author and her research teams; more independent testing of the DA is needed, as is further assessment of the instrument according to specific ethnic and cultural groups. In addition, protective actions of victims or of the system cannot be taken into account with the DA. Ellen Pence's Community Safety Audit system has promise for assessing the protections that the community has in place for abuse victims.

Another system that has potential for lethality risk assessment is the threat assessment system, DV MOSAIC (de Becker & Associates, 2000). This computerized method of assessing threat in IPV cases was developed based on domestic violence (DV) homicide cases and has advantages in that many of the individual protective factors are built into the factors assessed. There is also an IQ score given that helps a practitioner identify if missing information is compromising his or her ability to make an accurate assessment.

In the RAVE study, DV MOSAIC was the most accurate of the four methods tested in identifying the risk of stalking (Campbell et al., 2005). However, DV MOSAIC is not an instrument in the conventional sense, and its predictive validity for IP homicide cannot be calculated using usual methods. In fact, determining the predictive validity of any lethality risk assessment is nearly impossible because of the difficulties outlined above (low base rates or rarity of occurrence, ethics, lack of accurate information about risk factors after a homicide). Therefore creative research strategies need to be further developed as well as risk assessments that better take into account the community safety context, the perceptions and protective actions of victims, as well as the history of abuse and dangerousness of the abuser.

CONCLUSIONS

It is not particularly useful to scare all battered women with dire predictions of homicide; neither is it ethically or legally responsible not to warn those in particular danger of their risk. Many abused women in serious danger are clearly able to identify their risk, but approximately half apparently will not (Nicolaidis, et al., 2003). The most difficult cases, of course, are those in which the degree of danger is not clearly apparent. It is also important to realize that some couples are mutually violent and will not present as the more usual battering pattern. These cases, too, can result in homicide (Campbell, 1992).

Should all cases in which abuse or mutual violence is detected be routinely assessed for homicide risk? Because abuse is such a serious risk factor for homicide between intimates, if the practitioner is working with a potential victim, the answer is yes. Even in cases in which the risk is apparently low, knowledge of risk factors for homicide can be used later by the potential victim in decision making if the violence escalates, as it frequently does, especially in cases of heightened risk.

When dealing with the abused partner, she (or much less often, he) should be an active participant in determining the degree of danger and what she should do next. The clinician can present the instrument or results of an assessment to the victim and discuss what risk factors are present and allow her to make her own decisions about future actions based on the assessment. Safety planning based on level of risk of homicide and addressed toward modifiable risk factors that are present is much more evidence-based practice than generic safety planning.

The risk is that the clinician becomes paternalistic and prescribes certain courses of action that have not been shown to be protective. Or that a victim, even when presented with the evidence of high risk, chooses not to take action to protect her-or himself. The clinician may decide to call in the criminal justice system regardless of the victim's choice, using a risk assessment with research support as the basis for such action. Or what is probably more justifiable, given preferences for client autonomy and empowerment, as well as the current state of knowledge, the practitioner can use the level of risk as a modifier of his or her assertiveness in safety planning, restricting but not eliminating choices presented to victims.

For instance, in situations of highest risk, a practitioner could present choices in terms of what might be done but not accept doing nothing. Practitioners in other systems should keep in mind that the wife abuse shelter network as well as the National Domestic Violence Hotline (1-800-799-SAFE) can be extremely helpful even if the victim is against actually going into the shelter.

TABLE 5.2   Risk Factors Identified Across Majority of Experts

Access to/ownership of guns

Use of weapon in prior abusive incidents

Threats with weapon(s) (gun, knife)

Threats to kill

Serious injury in prior abusive incidents

Threats of suicide

Drug or alcohol abuse

Forced sex of female partner

Possessiveness/extreme jealousy/extreme dominance

As with most areas of violence, spousal homicide presents the dilemma of clinicians being caught between having both an ethical and a legal mandate to do accurate prediction without an unerring means of doing so. However, we have some consistent information about risk factors. Table 5.2 is a list of risk factors (over and above prior domestic violence) identified by the majority of the experts in the field, including those on the Danger Assessment. All clinicians working with battered women and their abusers, whether in the mental health or physical health systems, the criminal justice system, or the shelter/advocacy system, at least owe their clients a discussion of these homicide risk factors.

NOTE

1. The Kuder Richardson formula is recommended to assess internal consistency for instruments such as the Danger Assessment that use nonweighted dichotomous responses (Knapp, 1991). When used with the Danger Assessment, however, it does increase the reliability coefficient more than a hundredth of a point and therefore is not reported.

Acknowledgments. Research reported in this chapter was supported by the National Institute for Drug Abuse (R01 DA/AA11156, J. Campbell, Principle Investigator), and the National Institute of Justice (2000WTVX0011, J. Campbell, Principle Investigator).

REFERENCES

Ægisdóttir, S., White, M. J., Spengler, P. M., Maugherman, A. S., Anderson, L. A., Cook, R. S., et al. (2006). The meta-analysis of clinical judgment project: Fifty-six years of accumulated research on clinical versus statistical prediction. *The Counseling Psychologist, 34,* 341–382.

Berk, R. A., Berk, S. F., Loseke, D. R., & Rauma, D. (1983). Mutual combat and other family violence myths. In D. Finkelhor, R. J. Gelles, G. T. Hotaling, & M. A. Straus (Eds.), *The dark side of families: Current family violence research* (pp. 197–212). Beverly Hills, CA: Sage.

Browne, A. (1987). *Battered women who kill.* New York: Free Press.

Campbell, J. C. (1981). Misogyny and homicide of women. *Advances in Nursing Science, 3*(2), 67–85.

Campbell, J. C. (1986). Assessment of risk of homicide for battered women. *Advances in Nursing Science, 8*(4), 36–51.

Campbell, J. C. (1992). "If I can't have you, no one can": Power and control in homicide of female partners. In J. Radford & D. Russell (Eds.), *Femicide: The politics of woman killing* (pp. 99–113). New York: Twayne.

Campbell, J. C. (Ed.) (1995). *Assessing dangerousness: Violence by sexual offenders, batterers, and child abusers.* Newbury Park, CA: Sage.

Campbell, J. C. (2004). Helping women understand their risk in situations of intimate partner violence. *Journal of Interpersonal Violence, 19*(12), 1464–1477.

Campbell, J. C. (2005). Assessing dangerousness in domestic violence cases: History, challenges and opportunities. *Criminology and Public Policy, 4,* 801–820.

Campbell, J. C., Miller, P., Cardwell, M., & Belknap, R. A. (1994). Relationship status of battered women over time. *Journal of Family Violence, 9,* 99–111.

Campbell, J. C., O'Sullivan, C., Roehl, J., & Webster, D. W. (2005). *Intimate partner violence risk assessment validation study:* The RAVE study. Final report to the National Institute of Justice. (NCJ 209731–209732). Retrieved January 8, 2007, from http://www.ncjrs.org/pdffiles1/nij/grants/209731.pdf

Campbell, J. C., O'Sullivan, C., Roehl, J., & Webster, D. W. (2007). *Assessing risk from violent intimate partners: The RAVE Study.* Research in Briefs. Washington, DC: National Institute of Justice.

Campbell, J. C., Rose, L. E., Kub, J., & Nedd, D. (1998). Voices of strength and resistance: A contextual and longitudinal analysis of women's responses to battering. *Journal of Interpersonal Violence, 13,* 743–762.

Campbell, J. C., Sharps, P. W., & Glass, N. E. (2001). Risk assessment for intimate partner homicide. In G. F. Pinard & L. Pagani (Eds.), *Clinical assessment of dangerousness: Empirical contributions* (pp. 136–157). New York: Cambridge University Press.

Campbell, J. C., Webster, D., & Glass, N. E. (in press). The Danger Assessment: Validation of a lethality risk assessment instrument for intimate partner femicide. *Journal of Interpersonal Violence.*

Campbell, J. C., Webster, D., Koziol-McLain, J., Block C. R., Campbell, D., Curry, M. A., et al. (2003). Risk factors for femicide in abusive relationships: Results from a multi-site case control study. *American Journal of Public Health, 93,* 1089–1097.

Centers for Disease Control and Prevention. (2001). *Ten leading causes of death.* Retrieved January 8, 2007, from http\\www.cdc.gov/nchs/data/dvs/LCWK2_2001.pdf

Daly, M., & Wilson, M. (1988). *Homicide.* Hawthorne, NY: Aldine.

de Becker, G., & Associates. (2000). *Domestic Violence Method (DV MOSAIC).* Retrieved September 18, 2006, from http://www.mosaicsystem.com/dv.htm

Department of Health and Human Services, Public Health Service (DHHS). (2000). *Healthy people 2010 Progress Report: Progress toward the national health promotion and disease prevention objectives.* Washington, DC: Government Printing Office.

Fagan, J. A., Stewart, D. K., & Hansen, K. V. (1983). Violent men or violent husbands? Background factors and situational correlates. In D. Finkelhor, R. J. Gelles, G. T. Hotaling, & M. A. Straus (Eds.), *The dark side of families: Current family violence research* (pp. 49–68). Beverly Hills, CA: Sage.

Fox, J. A., & Zawitz, M. W. (2004). *Homicide trends in the United States.* Washington, DC: U.S. Department of Justice, Bureau of Justice Statistics.

Goodman, L. A., Dutton, M. A., & Bennett, L. (2000). Predicting repeat abuse among arrested batterers. *Journal of Interpersonal Violence, 15,* 63–74.

Hart, B. (1988). Beyond the "duty to warn": A therapist's "duty to protect" battered women and children. In K. Yllo & M. Bograd (Eds.), *Feminist perspectives on wife abuse* (pp. 234–248). Newbury Park, CA: Sage.

Heckert, D. A., & Gondolf, E. W. (2004). Battered women's perceptions of risk versus risk factors and instruments in predicting repeat reassault. *Journal of Interpersonal Violence, 19,* 778–800.

Hilton, N. Z., Harris, G. T., & Rice, M. E. (2006). Sixty-six years of research on clinical versus actuarial prediction of violence. *The Counseling Psychologist, 34,* 400–409.

Hudson, W., & McIntosh, S. (1981). The index of spouse abuse. *Journal of Marriage and the Family, 43*(4), 873–888.

Johnson, M. P. (in press). Conflict and control: Gender, symmetry, and asymmetry in domestic violence. *Violence Against Women.*

Joint Commission on the Accreditation of Healthcare Organizations. (2006). *Accreditation manual for hospitals.* Chicago, IL: Author.

Jurik, N. C., & Winn, R. (1990). Gender and homicide: A comparison of men and women who kill. *Violence and Victims, 5,* 227–242.

Knapp, T. R. (1991). Focus on psychometrics-coefficient alpha: Conceptualizations and anomalies. *Research in Nursing and Health, 14,* 157–460.

Koziol-McLain, J., Webster, D., McFarlane, J., Block, C. R., Ulrich, Y., Glass, N., et al. (2006). Risk factors for femicide-suicide in abusive relationships: Results from a multi-site case control study. *Violence and Victims, 21,* 3–21.

Langford, L., Isaac, N. E., & Kabat, S. (1998). Homicides related to intimate partner violence in Massachusetts. *Homicide Studies, 2*(4), 353–377.

Lilienthal, C. (2004). Settlement in action in Pike County. *Pennsylvania Law Weekly, 27*(52), 1, 14.

Mann, C. R. (1990). Black female homicide in the United States. *Journal of Interpersonal Violence, 5,* 176–201.

McClane, G. E., Strack, G. B., & Hawley, D. (2001). Violence: Recognition, management, and prevention: A review of 300 attempted strangulation cases. Part II: Clinical evaluation of the surviving victim. *The Journal of Emergency Medicine, 21*(3), 311–315.

McFarlane, J., Parker, B., Soeken, K., & Bullock, L. (1992). Assessing for abuse during pregnancy: Severity and frequency of injuries and associated entry into prenatal care. *Journal of the American Medical Association, 267,* 3176–3178.

Mercy, J. A., & Saltzman, L. E. (1989). Fatal violence among spouses in the United States, 1976–85. *American Journal of Public Health, 79,* 595–599.

Miller, M., & Morris, N. (1988). Predictions of dangerousness: An argument for limited use. *Violence and Victims, 3*(4), 263–283.

Moracco, K. E., Runyan, C. W., & Butts, J. D. (1998). Femicide in North Carolina. *Homicide Studies, 2,* 422–446.

Morton, E., Runyan, C. W., Moracco, K. E., & Butts, J. D. (1998). Partner homicide-suicide involving female homicide victims: A population-based study in North Carolina, 1998–1992. *Violence and Victims, 13*(2), 91–106.

Nicolaidis, C., Curry, M. A., McFarlane, J., Ulrich, Y., Koziol-McLain, J., & Campbell, J. C. (2003). Could we have known? A qualitative analysis of data from women who survived an attempted homicide by an intimate partner. *General Internal Medicine, 18,* 788–794.

Pinard, G. F., & Pagani, L. (Eds.) (2001). *Clinical assessment of dangerousness: Empirical contributions.* New York: Cambridge University Press.

Sharps, P. W., Campbell, J. C., Campbell, D. W., Gary, F. A., & Webster, D. (2001). The role of alcohol use in intimate partner femicide. *The American Journal on Addictions, 10,* 122–135.

Sharps, P. W., Koziol-McLain, J., Campbell, J. C., McFarlane, J., Sachs, C. J., & Xu, X. (2001). Health care providers' missed opportunities for preventing femicide. *Preventive Medicine, 33,* 373–380.

Small, L. B. (1985). Psychotherapists' duty to warn: Ten years after Tarasoff. *Golden Gate University Law Review, 15*(2), 271–300.

Sonkin, D. J., Martin, D., & Walker, L. E. (1985). *The male batterer: A treatment approach.* New York: Springer Publishing.

Straus, M. A., & Gelles, R. J. (1990). *Physical violence in American families: Risk factors and adaptions to violence in 8,145 families.* New Brunswick, NJ: Transaction Books.

Straus, M. J. (1991, November). *Severity and chronicity of domestic assault: Measurement implications for criminal justice intervention.* Paper presented at the Annual American Society of Chriminology Conference , San Francisco

Stuart, E. P., & Campbell, J. C. (1989). Assessment of patterns of dangerousness with battered women. *Issues in Mental Health Nursing, 10,* 245–260.

Wadman, M. C., & Muelleman, R. (1999). Domestic violence homicides: ED use before victimization. *American Journal of Emergency Medicine, 17*(7), 689–691.

Weisz, A. N., Tolman, R. M., & Saunders, D. G. (2000). Assessing the risk of severe domestic violence: The importance of survivors' predictions. *Journal of Interpersonal Violence, 15,* 75–90.

Wilson, M. (1991, November). *Problems in defining marital-like relationships.* Paper presented at the meetings of the American Society of Criminology, San Francisco.

CHAPTER 6

Assessing Risk of Intimate Partner Violence

N. Zoe Hilton and Grant T. Harris

Violence against intimate partners has existed over centuries (e.g., Hilton, 1989) and in most societies (Levinson, 1989), and even among many nonhuman species (Lalumière, Harris, Quinsey, & Rice, 2005). Only since the latter twentieth century has it been widely viewed as a serious social, criminal, and public health problem. Nearly half a million women victims of partner violence seek treatment for injuries each year in the United States (Rennisen & Welchans, 2000), more than for any other cause of injury to women (Stark & Flitcraft, 1996). Many more seek clinical interventions for mental health effects including posttraumatic stress disorder, depression, and substance abuse (e.g., Logan, Walker, Jordan, & Leukefeld, 2006).

Innovations in criminal justice responses to partner assault have expanded rapidly in the past decade (e.g., Buzawa & Buzawa, 2003; Hilton & Harris, in press), building on earlier attention to the limited and sometimes counterproductive effects of traditional approaches. More recently, gender-neutral interventions have also been criticized for failing to identify the primary aggressor (e.g., Landau, 2000; Martin, 1997). In fact, although contemporary policies on intimate partner violence (IPV) often aim for gender neutrality, almost all research on the risk of IPV has been concerned with male offenders and female victims. As such, it cannot necessarily be applied directly to female offenders or to same-sex relationships. In this chapter, where some information is known about both male and female perpetrators of violence (which is most often true in college or community studies) we will use the term IPV. When knowledge is limited to male-to-female violence in marital or cohabiting relationships (usually from criminal justice or treatment studies) we will refer to wife assault.

There has been an increasing trend for forensic clinicians, who traditionally assess risk of violence in general, to predict domestic violence specifically. Decision makers are also becoming interested not only in who will be violent toward a partner, but how soon and how severely. Furthermore, IPV is somewhat unique in that it is not only traditional assessors but also courts, police, victim services, nurses, crisis counselors, and even victims themselves, who are expected to assess the risk of IPV and intervene where necessary. In this chapter, then, we will review not only standard procedures for predicting IPV that have been published since the turn of this century, but also risk markers and variables that may have some predictive usefulness where such a standardized procedure is unavailable. We will also highlight the Ontario Domestic Assault Risk Assessment (ODARA), a validated actuarial risk assessment tool that can be used by front-line assessors from a variety of offender- and victim-service sectors, and discuss some of the practical issues in assessing the risk of IPV: intuitive versus statistical prediction, ethical concerns, and risk communication.

RISK MARKERS AND PREDICTORS

In the first edition of this volume, Saunders (1995) noted that few longitudinal studies of intimate partner violence existed. A longitudinal research study would measure characteristics of perpetrators, victims, and circumstances at one time and then repeat the measurements at a later time to ascertain who experiences repeated violence. Such follow-up research is best able to establish truly predictive connections between various characteristics and repeated violence, and thereby inform hypotheses about the actual causes of violence. In the absence of follow-up research, Saunders (1995) discussed "risk markers" rather than predictors. Extensive research attempting to identify risk markers—characteristics that distinguish men who assault their wives from those who do not—has been conducted by sampling known wife assaulters, perusing criminal records databases, and surveying college students or members of the general population (see reviews by Buzawa and Buzawa, 2003; and Hilton & Harris, 2005).

Risk of Assault in Previously Nonviolent Couples

The first generation of research into the correlates of intimate partner violence identified variables at the level of childhood experience, adult adjustment, and socioeconomic status, similar to studies of the correlates of violent behavior in general. For example, lower income, common-law marriage, and ethnic minority status appear to be risk markers for self- and partner-reports of IPV (e.g., Aldarondo & Sugarman, 1996; Brownridge & Halli, 2001; Caetano, Field, Ramisetty-Mikler, & McGrath, 2005; Cattaneo & Goodman, 2005; Torres et al., 2000). Criminal acts, whether detected or undetected, property or violent offenses, are also more likely among perpetrators of IPV in marital and dating relationships (e.g., Ramirez, 2005; Straus & Ramirez, 2004). A large study of wife assaulters in institutional or community treatment revealed that severely abusive men scored higher on many psychological risk markers such as anger, hostility, depression, and antisociality than less abusive men whose scores, in turn, were higher than nonabusive men from the same samples (Hanson, Cadsky, Harris, & Lalonde, 1997). Studies of clinical characteristics have added jealousy, insecure attachment, poor assertiveness, and attitudes supportive of interpersonal violence (e.g., Holtzworth-Munroe, Bates, Smutzler, & Sandin, 1997). Psychiatric history appears not to be a risk marker (e.g., Hanson et al., 1997). Although controversial because of its potential to be used as an excuse, alcohol abuse has proven to be especially good at distinguishing severe wife assaulters and those with antisocial personality characteristics (Murphy, O'Farrell, Fals-Stewart, & Feehan, 2001; Sharps, Campbell, Campbell, Foy, & Webster, 2001; Thompson & Kingree, 2006).

Self-reports of witnessing parental violence or experiencing physical abuse are more likely among IPV perpetrators in community, treatment, and inmate samples (Dutton & Hart, 1992; O'Leary & Curley, 1986; Straus, 1983; see review and discussion in Hines & Saudino, 2002). Men's exposure to violence in childhood has also been linked to aggression in college dating relationships, and domineering behavior in the laboratory (Skuja & Halford, 2004). A recent study of the intergenerational transmission of IPV among identical and fraternal twins found that genetic relatedness accounted for similarity in both psychological and physical IPV (Hines & Saudino, 2004). Thus, parental IPV or child abuse is a risk marker for IPV, but the mechanism might be primarily via common inheritance rather than social modeling, for example.

Risk markers identified in correlational research have revealed candidate variables for attempts to predict IPV even among individuals not already identified as violent. Dutton (1995) developed the 29-item self-report Propensity for Abusiveness Scale (PAS) based on associations among men's childhood and adult adjustment variables and their female partners' reports of IPV. Items include measures of anger, trauma symptoms, parental treatment, and attachment style with borderline personality features. Scores on the PAS for wife assaulters, in clinical and nonclinical samples, have been associated with partner reports of threats and physical aggression (Dutton, Landolt, Starzomski, & Bodnarchuk, 2001).

There have now been a few longitudinal prediction studies of the onset of IPV, conducted by assessing men who are not yet maritally violent, and following up several years later to obtain self- or partner-reports of assault. In one large study of young couples, men's self-reports of parental violence and attitudes toward violence before marriage were associated with later wife assault; in contrast, self-reports of actual violence to family members and peers in youth were unrelated to wife assault (O'Leary, Malone, & Tyree, 1994). In another study, childhood exposure to violence was a predictor of IPV, but it appeared to be a weaker predictor than conduct disorder (Ehrensaft et al., 2003). Longitudinal research has consistently confirmed the importance of alcohol use, which predicts IPV among newlyweds even after controlling for premarital aggression (e.g., Heyman, O'Leary, & Jouriles, 1995; Leonard & Senchak, 1996), and which increases verbal conflict in both violent and non-violent couples (Leonard & Roberts, 1998).

In summary, there is a small amount of true prediction research on the risk factors that would identify which men will eventually engage in IPV. Those interested in assessing the risk of IPV in such men should attend to parental violence, conduct disorder, substance abuse (primarily alcohol), psychological aggression and conflict, personality disorder (especially antisocial), mood disorder, anger and hostility, certain attitudes supportive of violence, and the level of appropriately assertive behavior (Hilton & Harris, 2005). The PAS might assist in this respect. It is important to distinguish here between IPV onset and IPV recidivism. Variables found to distinguish wife assaulters from nonassaulters will not necessarily be useful in determining which wife assaulters will commit the most severe or prolific subsequent assaults. Parental violence, for example, is a strong risk factor for the onset of wife assault, but has not been found to predict IPV recidivism (Aldarondo & Sugarman, 1996; Hanson & Wallace-Capretta, 2004). Longitudinal research has found that assault early in a relationship, particularly acts of minor violence, could be a one-time event (O'Leary et al., 1989; Quigley & Leonard, 1996). Men who re-assault severely or frequently exhibit more extreme scores on predictor variables than less severe or one-time recidivists (Gondolf, 2002, Chapter 8; Hanson & Wallace-Capretta, 2004). This finding suggests that it might be worth using predictors of repeated IPV for the early identification of men at risk for wife assault.

Risk of Repeated Assault Among Wife Assaulters

Since the first edition of this volume, progress has been made in identifying valid indicators of the risk of IPV recidivism. As with work in the correlates of

IPV, the most consistent predictors are similar to predictors of general criminal and violent recidivism: younger age, lower socioeconomic status, marital
conflict, verbal abuse, severity of wife assault history, and arrest history for
domestic violence (e.g., Aldarondo & Sugarman, 1996; Bennett, Goodman,
& Dutton, 2000; Benson, Fox, DeMaris, & VanWyk, 2003; Foa, Cascardi,
Zoellner, & Feeny, 2000; Gondolf, 2002; Jacobson, Gottman, Gortner, Berns,
& Shortt, 1996; Jasinksi, 2001; O'Leary et al., 1994; Quigley & Leonard,
1996). Men who commit IPV and who also commit other violent or antisocial
acts have consistently been identified as being at especially high risk of recidivism (see reviews by Marshall & Holtzworth-Munroe, 2002; and Monson
& Langhinrichsen-Rohling, 1998). Hanson and Wallace-Capretta (2004) reported that perpetrator age and score on the Level of Service Inventory (a risk
assessment for criminal recidivism) were sufficient to predict repeated assault
against intimate partners.

The adequate assessment of the risk of subsequent IPV among known wife
assaulters, then, requires knowledge of past aggression and antisocial behavior, including alcohol consumption. In a prospective study of men in a wife
assault treatment program, both self- and partner-reports of alcohol use and
physical aggression were obtained each day; men's drinking was associated
with a large increase in the occurrence of assaults the same day, especially
among alcoholics (Fals-Stewart, 2003). Huss and Langhinrichsen-Rohling
(2000) illustrated the similarities between the characteristics of the most serious wife assaulters (antisociality, both severe IPV and general violence, low
physiological arousal, substance abuse, resistance to treatment) and the traits
typically associated with psychopathy (see Hare, 2003). Psychopaths exhibit
glibness, proneness to boredom, unempathic callousness, and a history of
early behavior problems, irresponsibility, impulsivity, and criminal versatil-
ity. In a study of men court-mandated to treatment for IPV, both substance
abuse and psychopathy were strongly associated with self-reported violence
(McBurnett et al., 2001). The gold standard for the assessment of psychopathy is the Hare Psychopathy Checklist (PCL-R) (Hare, 1991, 2003). PCL-R
score tends to be lower among wife assaulters than among violent offenders in
general, but recent studies indicate that it may be one of the strongest predictors of wife assault recidivism (Grann & Wedin, 2002; Hilton, Harris, & Rice,
2001) and can improve upon existing assessment tools for domestic violence
dangerous behavior (Hilton, Harris, Rice, Houghton, & Eke, in press).

Recent research has indicated that the victim herself can assess the risk
of repeated assault by her partner (e.g., Weisz, Tolman, & Saunders, 2000)
and her concern about future assaults is strong enough to outperform such
conventional predictors as jealousy, injury, and the use of weapons (Hilton,
Harris, Rice, Lang, Cormier, & Lines, 2004). Women's perceptions of safety

and of the likelihood of wife assault recidivism predicted multiple reassault (Gondolf, 2002). Fear might reflect a history of severe assault, itself a predictor of recidivism, or it might increase recall of past assaults. Thus, women's own predictions are relevant to the assessment of the risk of wife assault recidivism.

Frequent and Severe Assault

As reviewed above, the strongest predictors of wife assault and its repetition also predict greater frequency and severity of wife assault. The presence of children, especially stepchildren, also increases both the risk and severity of wife assault recidivism (Hilton et al., 2004). Researchers examining lethal assaults in the population have observed similar associations, such as female victims being of childbearing age (controlling for husband's age), and having children from a previous partner, which have been interpreted as evidence for male jealousy and proprietary behavior (e.g., Shackelford, Buss, and Peters, 2000; Shackelford, Buss, & Weekes-Shackelford, 2003; Wilson & Daly, 1998). Research comparing abused women in nonlethal and lethal cases supports this interpretation; having a child from a previous partner and ending the relationship for a new sexual partner have been reported to be risk factors for lethal assault (Campbell, Webster, & Koziol-McLain, 2003). The overlapping ability of most predictors to predict wife assault overall as well as its frequency and severity, including lethal assault, supports the suggestion that assessors exclusively concerned with the risk of lethal assault should nevertheless attend to scores on a valid risk assessment for overall wife assault recidivism. Such instruments, particularly if designed for brief, frontline use, could be used in all cases being assessed for the risk of wife assault. Then, in relatively high-scoring cases, particular attention could be paid to unique events in the relationship that are associated with lethality, such as those assessed by the Danger Assessment (see Chapter 5, this volume).

Predicting Assault After Intervention

Treatment programs for wife assaulters emerged soon after wife assault became a public issue and quickly became very popular, with court-mandated treatment being a common aspect of sentencing or diversion (e.g., Hamberger & Hastings, 1993; Hilton & Harris, in press). Unfortunately, few treatment evaluations have included a suitable comparison group, and despite debate over appropriate treatment models (e.g., psycho-educational, cognitive behavioral) no evaluation has demonstrated that one reduces recidivism more than any other, or more than no intervention. In their meta-analysis, Babcock,

Green, and Robie (2004) found only five scientifically sound studies comparing treatment with a nontreatment control group, and, in the aggregate, a minimal effect of treatment on wife assault recidivism.

In treatment evaluation studies, it is important to compare the outcomes of those men exposed to treatment to a comparable group not exposed. Moving cases who drop out of treatment, those who refuse, and those rejected as unsuitable to the comparison group, confounds the treatment effect with the effect of the perpetrator's motivation, compliance, and preexisting risk of recidivism (Rice & Harris, 2003). In this way, an apparent effect of treatment might actually be caused by the attrition of participants who represented the highest pretreatment risk of recidivism—perhaps especially psychopaths (Huss, Covell, & Langhinrichsen-Rohling, 2006). Research into the role of treatment as a moderator of risk has not yet provided much basis for optimism. Hanson and Wallace-Capretta (2004) failed to find significant correlations between recidivism and posttreatment improvement in substance abuse, attitudes, and relationship variables among men in treatment for wife assault. In this study, treatment did not contribute to the prediction of recidivism. In two recent studies of wife assaulters identified in police records of domestic assault (Hilton & Harris, 2005) or assessed by probation officers (Williams & Houghton, 2004), having had treatment was actually associated with greater likelihood of recidivism. Of course, treatment participation might be an index of higher pretreatment risk because treatment might be more often mandated for serious or repeat assaulters than for other offenders. Again, interpretation is hampered by lack of information about untreated men and dropouts, but it is clear that, other factors being equal, there is no empirical basis for considering a man to be at lower risk for committing wife assault by virtue of his having participated in treatment.

Risk Factors for Treatment Attrition

Despite the lack of evidence in favor of using treatment participation in assessing risk, assessors can get important information from treatment records. Treatment attrition is itself a predictor of recidivism. For example, in a study of wife assaulters on probation, about half of whom were court-mandated to treatment (in this case, men with fewer prior convictions) the treatment mandate itself was not associated with recidivism (Gordon & Moriarty, 2003); instead, recidivism was associated with less participation, and also with socioeconomic and antisociality variables typically associated with increased recidivism (i.e., lower income and education, prior domestic violence convictions, substance abuse). Several studies have shown that most men dropped out of treatment, and dropouts were more likely than completers to recidivate

(Babcock & Steiner, 1999; Cadsky, Hanson, Crawford, & Lalonde, 1996; Shepard, Falk, & Elliott, 2002). Furthermore, dropout was predicted by variables that also predict wife assault recidivism: denial of problems, younger age, criminal history, hostility, substance abuse, and lifestyle instability, as well as the severity of violence history (e.g., Dalton, 2001; Daly & Pelowski, 2000; Daly, Power, & Gondolf, 2001; Hanson & Wallace-Capretta, 2004; Rooney & Hanson, 2001), all variables also known to be associated with violent recidivism in general (e.g., Quinsey, Harris, Rice, & Cormier, 2006).

Probation officers' ratings of wife assaulters' cooperation, responsibility, and treatment motivation were not associated with treatment completion (Babcock & Steiner, 1999); nor were men's self-reports of perceived likelihood and severity of consequences for quitting, self-esteem, social support, stress, and marital relations (Heckert & Gondolf, 2000; Tutty, Bidgood, Rothery, & Bidgood, 2001). In research with sex offenders in treatment, those who received favorable reports from therapists were most likely to recidivate (Seto & Barbaree, 1999). Thus, clinical ratings of treatment progress should not be used in risk assessment.

PREDICTION TOOLS

Risk Assessments for IPV

There are many risk assessments created on an ad hoc, rational basis, and used in various North American jurisdictions, but most have not been published in the peer reviewed literature (Roehl & Guertin, 2000). Evaluations are rare, and some yield poor predictive accuracy (e.g., K-SID; Heckert & Gondolf, 2004). Predictive accuracy of a risk assessment is its ability to discriminate between recidivists and nonrecidivists. The accuracy of a risk assessment can be indexed by a variety of statistics. Some, such as hit rates and false positives, percentage agreement, and correlation, can fluctuate with the base rate of recidivism in the study sample. The preferred statistic, ROC area under the curve, is much less dependent on the base rate, and reflects the tradeoff between sensitivity (hit rate or ability to detect recidivists) and the specificity (avoidance of false alarms or ability to predict nonrecidivists) across the range of scores on the assessment (Rice & Harris, 1995, 2005). ROC area ranges from 0 to 1.0, where 1.0 represents perfect prediction, 0.5 represents no prediction, and 0 represents perfect inverse prediction.

The Domestic Violence Screening Instrument (DVSI) has been published along with scoring instructions and validation data (Williams & Grant, 2006; Williams & Houghton, 2004). This 12-item tool includes items reflecting domestic violence history, treatment for domestic violence or substance abuse, and the current offense, particularly regarding restraining orders. In a large sample of arrested wife assaulters, the DVSI scored by probation officers significantly predicted subsequent wife assault arrests up to 18 months later (ROC area = .60, Williams & Houghton, 2004).

The Danger Assessment (DA; Chapter 5, this volume), although intended to assess an abused woman's risk of lethal assault, has also been studied for its ability to predict wife assault recidivism overall. Weisz et al. (2000) interviewed women whose partners had recently been convicted of domestic assault, and scored most of the DA items. Total score on these items made a small but statistically significant contribution to a multivariate analysis predicting new incidents of assault or serious threats up to four months later, as measured in a second interview. In a similar study with a three-month follow-up, Goodman, Dutton, and Bennett (2000) reported that a high DA score significantly increased the odds of new assaults and threats, even when controlling for extent of prior violence. The predictive accuracy of the DA in follow-up studies has been supported when scored from offender file review (ROC = .64, Hilton et al., 2004) and victim interview (ROC = .70, Heckert & Gondolf, 2004).

To date, the most-tested clinical assessment specifically for assessing the risk of IPV is the Spousal Assault Risk Assessment (SARA; e.g., Kropp & Hart, 2000). The SARA was designed as a set of guidelines for assessors of family violence. Its 20 items, each scored 0–2, include some childhood history and adult criminal and antisocial history variables as well as other indicators of psychological adjustment, and items pertaining to spousal assault specifically. Some items are clearly related to the empirical research literature on the predictors of IPV or recidivism, whereas others were selected on the basis of clinical experience, with the aim of creating an assessment that is based upon empirical research but also consistent with users' opinions. The SARA requires scoring each item, noting the number of items present, and judging whether any item is critical, followed by a summary clinical judgment of the risk of imminent or other future harm to family members (Kropp, Hart, Webster, & Eaves, 1999, pp. 9–10). In the first published test of the SARA, the total score did not distinguish recidivists from other wife assaulters, but the summary risk rating—primarily a clinical judgment—did yield a statistically significant relationship (Kropp & Hart, 2000). In subsequent studies, total score has been reported to be related to wife assault recidivism (ROC areas of .65, Grann & Wedin, 2002; .67, Hilton et al., 2004; .64, Heckert & Gondolf, 2004; .65, Williams & Houghton, 2004).

Actuarial risk assessments for violence, and for wife assault in particular, have shown greater predictive accuracy than other assessment tools

(Ægisdóttir et al., 2006; Grann & Wedin, 2002; Hilton et al., 2004; Hilton, Harris, Rice, Houghton, & Eke, in press). Actuarial risk assessments are created on the basis of follow-up studies measuring the independent contribution of several variables to the prediction of the outcome; in this case, subsequent wife assault. Predictor items can be selected based on incremental validity—the extent to which each item adds to the predictive accuracy of those already selected. Each range of scores on the assessment is then related to an actuarial table; in this case, the likelihood of wife assault recidivism. The Ontario Domestic Assault Risk Assessment (ODARA; Hilton et al., 2004) is the first actuarial risk assessment constructed specifically for wife assault. The ODARA was designed to be a brief assessment for such frontline users as police officers and victim service providers. Its 13 dichotomous items were derived from information available to, and usually recorded by, police officers responding to domestic violence calls involving male perpetrators and female partners. The items cover domestic and nondomestic criminal history, threats and acts of confinement committed during the most recent incident, substance abuse, victim concern about future assaults, and other circumstances. These items were selected from many other potential predictors, using multivariate analyses and bootstrapping to maximize the likelihood that the ODARA would generalize to new samples. When constructed with cases identified in police reports, the ODARA yielded a large predictive accuracy (ROC area of .77) for wife assault recidivism, greater than reported for any other risk assessment that does not include the PCL-R. It maintained its accuracy on cross-validation (i.e., a replication with new cases not used in construction; ROC area of .72, Hilton et al., 2004). Scores on the ODARA are also related to the frequency, severity, and rapidity of wife assault recidivism (Hilton et al., 2004). Because the ODARA is an actuarial instrument, an individual's score can be compared to an actuarial table that indicates the rate of wife assault recidivism by perpetrators with the same score. These norms also indicate how men with each score compare with other known wife assaulters with respect to the risk of recidivism; that is, the norms indicate a perpetrator's rank order with respect to risk. Police officers and other users exhibit very high interrater agreement scoring real cases from records (Hilton et al., 2004).

Another actuarial tool, designed for the assessment of the risk of violent recidivism in general, the Violence Risk Appraisal Guide (VRAG; Quinsey et al., 2006), was reported to predict recidivism by wife assaulters, and more accurately than some risk assessments specifically for IPV (ROC areas of .75, Grann & Wedin, 2002; Hilton et al., 2001). The 12-item VRAG, which includes the PCL-R, was developed and first cross-validated on violent offenders from a maximum security institution, and has since been found to predict violent recidivism in more than 25 independent psychiatric and forensic samples (http://www.mhcp-research.com/ragreps.htm), including women (Harris, Rice, & Camilleri, 2004). Using the same empirical construction techniques as for the VRAG, we (Hilton, Harris, Rice, Houghton, & Eke, in press) created a similar, in-depth risk assessment for predicting wife assault recidivism by wife assaulters, the Domestic Violence Risk Appraisal Guide (DVRAG). Its 14 items, 13 similar to the ODARA, plus PCL-R score, are weighted in accordance with their individual predictive accuracy. In construction and cross-validation using samples of men undergoing probation assessment, the DVRAG had greater predictive accuracy than all other assessments tested. Because it requires more extensive knowledge of the offender's background and adjustment than does the ODARA, the DVRAG requires considerable time, well-researched psychosocial history, and training. The benefit is that, in a population of wife assaulters of higher than average risk, the DVRAG permits greater discrimination among perpetrators. For most wife assault assessment cases, and especially in frontline assessment situations, the ODARA yields an accurate prediction of wife assault recidivism with a shorter, simpler procedure.

Table 6.1 shows the average performance in all the published replication follow-up studies (of which we were aware) for total scores on the formal risk assessments discussed in this chapter. Although not intended as a meta-analysis (such an effort is underway; R. K. Hanson, 2007, personal communication), the number of studies and cases presented do permit the following tentative conclusions:

TABLE 6.1   Formal Instruments That Might Be Used to Assess the Risk of Wife Assault Recidivism

Instrument	First published	Mean ROC area	Studies (total N)	Notes
DA	2000	.62	5 (2696)	
DVRAG	—	.70	1 (346)	PCL-R required
DVSI	2004	.56	2 (1431)	
ODARA	2004	.67[a]	3 (837)	
SARA	2000	.62	6 (2361)	
VRAG	1993	.68[b]	2 (737)	PCL-R required

Note: DA = Danger Assessment; DVRAG = Domestic Violence Risk Appraisal Guide; DVSI = Domestic Violence Screening Instrument; ODARA = Ontario Domestic Assault Risk Assessment; SARA = Spousal Assault Risk Assessment; VRAG = Violence Risk Appraisal Guide.
[a].71 if actuarial construction sample is included ($n = 589$)
[b].69 if subsample of actuarial construction sample is included ($n = 80$)
First published refers to year of first peer-reviewed publication of predictive accuracy; Mean ROC area refers to predicting dichotomous domestic violence recidivism; Studies (total N) refers to the number of studies and cases in replication follow-up studies.

1. Actuarial assessments (VRAG, ODARA, DVRAG) perform better than those based on other methods.
2. Having been developed specifically for domestic violence does not guarantee a test's superior accuracy; scores on the VRAG appear to outperform those on the DA, DVSI, and SARA.
3. Domestic violence recidivism, as a subset of violent recidivism overall, is harder to predict. Mean ROC areas in Table 6.1 are lower, for example, than have been reported on average for the VRAG's prediction of violent recidivism in general.

Reduction of Wife Assault Through Arrest

There have been few good, controlled studies of the effect of criminal justice intervention on IPV. The criminal justice system is more concerned with service provision than demonstrable results, and outcomes are rarely rigorously evaluated (Hilton & Harris, in press). A notable exception is research on the effect of arrest across the United States in the 1980s and 1990s. The first study randomly assigned misdemeanor cases of wife assault to arrest or to other interventions and found that arrest was associated with the least recidivism (Sherman & Berk, 1984). Subsequent studies had difficulty replicating this effect, or reported that it depended on the length of follow-up, perpetrator characteristics, or the source of recidivism data (see review by Garner, Fagan, & Maxwell, 1995). More recently, we reported that police officers were more likely to arrest men who represented relatively high risk (based on ODARA scores), and when police and courts were aware of the perpetrators' risk scores they were also more likely to detain higher-risk perpetrators before trial (Hilton, Harris, & Rice, in press). Because interventions tend to be applied roughly in accordance with risk, the independent benefit of an intervention is difficult to assess, but it appears that arrest has a small effect in delaying recidivism (Garner, 1997), especially among lower-risk men (Hilton, Harris, & Rice in press).

PRACTICE ISSUES

The Role of Clinical Judgment

It is well established that actuarial methods of assessment are more accurate than unaided clinical judgment, especially in the appraisal of violence risk (Ægisdóttir et al., 2006; Grove & Meehl, 1996; Grove, Zald, Lebow, Snitz, & Nelson, 2000; Hilton, Harris, & Rice, 2006; Quinsey et al., 2006). That is, actuarial methods of selecting and combining risk factors to derive an estimate of offenders' risk of violent recidivism are consistently more valid than relying on assessors' experience, memory, familiarity with relevant research, and intuition. There is no evidence that blending assessors' clinical judgment with actuarial scores improves the accuracy achieved by actuarial methods alone (Quinsey et al., 2006). There is, however, an important role for clinical judgment in risk assessment. Many of the most valid risk-related items require clinical skill to evaluate (e.g., personality disorder, addictions, childhood history of aggression, and especially psychopathy). Clinical judgment should be used within the assessment tool rather than as an intuitive alternative to the statistical approach.

As described earlier, item selection for actuarial instruments is based on follow-up research that identifies the strongest empirical predictors of violent outcomes; the best predictors are selected first and further items are added only when they increase predictive accuracy. Despite the statistical methods used to construct actuarial instruments, the resulting assessment can be straightforward to interpret. The development and scoring process actually eliminates much of the human effort (and accompanying normal errors and biases) needed to process case information. Thus, some information (e.g., jealousy), although a valid predictor of recidivism, need not necessarily be evaluated because it is correlated with stronger predictors (e.g., threats of violence or victim fear). In addition, we have found that a wide range of users can score the ODARA with good reliability even without training, although they are significantly better after a one-day workshop (Hilton, Harris, Rice, Eke, & Lowe-Wetmore, 2006). Actuarial assessments tend to yield better interrater reliability than other, nonactuarial methods, so to the extent that poor reliability limits accuracy, actuarial tools are more likely to yield accurate assessments in practice. It is important to note that, no matter how an assessment is constructed, users have to address generalization to their own population. For example, a tool developed to predict IPV by men must be evaluated for IPV by women before it can be used to predict women's recidivism.

Ethical Concerns

As in most forensic domains concerning violent, criminal behavior, the assessment of the risk of IPV entails balancing perpetrators' civil rights against the right of potential victims to be free from criminal violence. Risk assessment is a tool to help decision makers examine that balance. It would make little sense to devote resources to distinguishing among perpetrators with respect to the risk of recidivism unless relevant decisions were made dependent on such distinctions. Thus, the point of conducting a risk assessment is to ensure that perpetrators identified as higher risk receive more incarceration, supervision, or treatment, for example, than those identified as lower risk. Likewise, the partners of perpetrators identified as higher risk should receive more intensive service (e.g., provision of phones directly linked to 911 service) than those identified as lower risk. In our view, it would be ethical to expend public resources on risk assessment in order to ensure differential case management overall and/or offender intervention as a result. Similarly, given that there is empirical information to permit valid distinctions among IPV cases with respect to the risk of recidivism, we regard it as an ethical obligation to ensure that the intensity and type of interventions be related to that risk, because any other way of apportioning resources (including treating all cases as equally dangerous) will result in avoidable subsequent violence, unnecessary loss of civil liberty, or both. For the same reason, we regard it as an ethical imperative to use the most accurate available means to assess the risk of IPV recidivism, irrespective of traditional professional models or the preferences of clinicians, lawyers, or commentators.

Risk Communication Among Agencies

In summarizing the literature on the risk of IPV, Saunders (1995) emphasized the need to disseminate this information to potential users, including police officers, who are not traditionally thought of as risk assessors. He also raised the question of whether offender programs and victims should share information. In our work with the ODARA, we collaborated with the Ontario Provincial Police to create an assessment that could be easily used by police officers and shared throughout the criminal justice system. We have also partnered with victim service providers to turn the ODARA into a victim interview format. During cross-sector risk assessment training sessions, participants have had the opportunity to learn about the ODARA together and to share ideas for communicating with each other about the risk posed by perpetrators, and faced by victims, in their respective services.

In traditional forensic assessment, though, research has demonstrated that clinicians tend to avoid the use of available actuarial assessments (e.g., Hilton, Harris, Rawson, & Beach, 2005; Hilton & Simmons, 1999) and the move toward clinician-friendly assessments has increased reliance on less accurate clinical judgment (Hilton, Harris, & Rice, 2006). There is an emerging research literature on how best to communicate violence risk assessment results in a way that results in improved decision making. We have found, for example, that forensic clinicians used risk-relevant case information to appraise risk in the absence of a numerical risk summary statement, but that providing a numerical statement improved risk communication (Hilton et al., 2005) whereas providing a nonnumerical statement (i.e., "low risk" or "high risk") had no beneficial effect (Hilton, Carter, Harris, & Sharpe, in press). Our research revealed that assessors disagreed substantially on the interpretation of such nonnumerical terms, and their nonnumerical evaluations were vulnerable to biases that impaired decision proficiency. In order for risk communication to be effective, then, and for offender and victim services to agree on the level of risk posed by any given perpetrator, they need to have a common language, but that "language" is most effectively expressed in numbers, including the likelihood of recidivism and comparison (rank order), which is given by actuarial tables.

SUMMARY

Attention to the assessment of the risk of IPV has increased dramatically in recent years, particularly regarding wife assault recidivism. Assessors should be aware of the striking similarity between the best predictors of IPV and the strongest predictors of general violence. This means that attempts to assess abused women's risk of being assaulted again should incorporate information about the perpetrator's criminal history and other measures of antisociality. Those who assess perpetrator risk should also attend to victim reports, because of recent studies indicating the value of the victim's concern for the future and of her assessment of her own risk. Thus, the need for communication of risk information among service providers is as valid today as it was over a decade ago (e.g., Saunders, 1995). Validated actuarial risk assessment tools are now available and can be used for effective risk assessment and communication.

REFERENCES

References marked with an asterisk were used to compute ROC areas in Table 6.1.

Ægisdóttir, S., White, M. J., Spengler, P. M., Maugherman, A. S., Anderson, L. A., Cook, R. S., et al. (2006). The meta-analysis of clinical judgment project: Fifty-six years of accumulated research on clinical versus statistical prediction. *The Counseling Psychologist, 34,* 341–382.

Aldarondo, E., & Sugarman, D. B. (1996). Risk marker analysis of the cessation and persistence of wife assault. *Journal of Consulting and Clinical Psychology, 64,* 1010–1019.

Babcock, J. C., Green, C. E., & Robie, C. (2004). Does batterers' treatment work? A meta-analytic review of domestic violence treatment. *Clinical Psychology Review, 23,* 1023–1053.

Babcock, J. C., & Steiner, R. (1999). The relationship between treatment, incarceration, and recidivism of battering: A program evaluation of Seattle's coordinated community response to domestic violence. *Journal of Family Psychology, 13,* 46–59.

Bennett, L., Goodman, L., & Dutton, M. A. (2000). Risk assessment among batterers arrested for domestic assault. *Violence Against Women, 6,* 1190–1203.

Benson, M. L., Fox, G. L., DeMaris, A., & Van Wyk, J. (2003). Neighborhood disadvantage, individual economic distress and violence against women in intimate relationships. *Journal of Quantitative Criminology, 19,* 207–235.

Brownridge, D. A., & Halli, S. S. (2001). *Explaining violence against women in Canada.* New York: Lexington Books.

Buzawa, E. S., & Buzawa, C. G. (2003). *Domestic violence: The criminal justice response.* Thousand Oaks, CA: Sage.

Cadsky, O., Hanson, R. K., Crawford, M., & Lalonde, C. (1996). Attrition from a male batterer treatment program: Client-treatment congruence and lifestyle instability. *Violence and Victims, 11,* 51–64.

Caetano, R., Field, C. A., Ramisetty-Mikler, S., & McGrath, C. (2005). The 5-year course of intimate partner violence among white, black, and Hispanic couples in the United States. *Journal of Interpersonal Violence, 20,* 1039–1057.

Campbell, J. C., Webster, D., & Koziol-McLain, J. (2003). Risk factors for femicide in abusive relationships: Results from a multisite case control study. *American Journal of Public Health, 93,* 1089–1097.

*Campbell, J. C., and others. RIB Final 11-151 [Jackie please provide full reference, thanks, Zoe]

Cattaneo, L. B., & Goodman, L. A. (2005). Risk factors for reabuse in intimate partner violence: A cross-disciplinary critical review. *Trauma, Violence and Abuse, 6,* 141–175.Levinson, D. (1989). *Family violence in cross-cultural perspective.* Newbury Park, CA: Sage.

Dalton, B. (2001). Batterer characteristics and treatment completion. *Journal of Interpersonal Violence, 16,* 1223–1238.

Daly, J. E., & Pelowski, S. (2000). Predictors of dropout among men who batter: A review of studies with implications for research and practice. *Violence and Victims, 15,* 137–160.

Daly, J. E., Power, T. G., & Gondolf, E. W. (2001). Predictors of batterer program attendance. *Journal of Interpersonal Violence, 16,* 971–991.

Dutton, D. G. (1995). A scale for measuring propensity for abusiveness. *Journal of Family Violence, 10,* 203–221.

Dutton, D. G., & Hart, S. D. (1992). Risk markers for family violence in a federally incarcerated population. *International Journal of Law and Psychiatry, 15,* 101–112.

Dutton, D. G., Landolt, M. A., Starzomski, A., & Bodnarchuk, M. (2001). Validation of the propensity for abusive scale in diverse male populations. *Journal of Family Violence, 16,* 59–73.

Ehrensaft, M. K., Cohen, P., Brown, J., Smailes, E., Chen, H., & Johnson, J. G. (2003). Intergenerational transmission of partner violence: A 20-year prospective study. *Journal of Consulting and Clinical Psychology, 71,* 741–753.

Fals-Stewart, W. (2003). The occurrence of partner physical aggression on days of alcohol consumption: A longitudinal diary study. *Journal of Consulting and Clinical Psychology, 71*, 41–52.

Foa, E. B., Cascardi, M., Zoellner, L. A., & Feeny, N. C. (2000). Psychological and environmental factors associated with partner violence. *Trauma, Violence, & Abuse, 1*, 67–91.

Garner, J. H. (1997). Evaluating the effectiveness of mandatory arrest for domestic violence in Virginia. *William & Mary Journal of Women and the Law, 3*, 223-240.

Garner, J. H., Fagan, J., & Maxwell, C. (1995). Published findings from the Spouse Assault Replication Program: A critical review. *Journal of Quantitative Criminology, 11*, 3-28.

Gondolf, E. W. (2002). *Batterer intervention systems.* Thousand Oaks, CA: Sage.

Goodman, L. A., Dutton, M. A., & Bennett, L. (2000). Predicting repeat abuse among arrested batterers. *Journal of Interpersonal Violence, 15*, 63–74.

Gordon, J. A., & Moriarty, L. J. (2003). The effects of domestic violence batterer treatment on domestic violence recidivism. *Criminal Justice and Behavior, 30*, 118–134.

*Grann, M., & Wedin, I. (2002). Risk factors for recidivism among spousal assault and spousal homicide offenders. *Psychology, Crime, and Law, 8*, 5–23.

Grove, W. M., & Meehl, P. E. (1996). Comparative efficiency of informal (subjective, impressionistic) and formal (mechanical, algorithmic) prediction procedures: The clinical-statistical controversy. *Psychology, Public Policy, and Law, 2*, 293–323.

Grove, W. M., Zald, D. H., Lebow, B. S., Snitz, B. E., & Nelson, C. (2000). Clinical versus mechanical prediction: A meta-analysis. *Psychological Assessment, 12*, 19 30.

Hamberger, L. K., & Hastings, J. E. (1993). Court-mandated treatment of men who assault their partner. In N. Z. Hilton (Ed.), *Legal responses to wife assault* (pp. 188–229). Newbury Park, CA: Sage.

Hanson, R. K., Cadsky, O., Harris, A., & Lalonde, C. (1997). Correlates of battering among 997 men: Family history, adjustment, and attitudinal differences. *Violence and Victims, 12*, 191–208.

Hanson, R. K., & Harris, A. (2000). Where should we intervene? Dynamic predictors of sex offense recidivism. *Criminal Justice and Behavior, 27*, 6–35.

Hanson, R. K., & Morton-Bourgon, K. (2004). *Predictors of sexual recidivism: An updated meta-analysis.* Public Safety and Emergency Preparedness Canada.

Hanson, R. T., & Wallace-Capretta, S. (2004). Predictors of criminal recidivism among male batterers. *Psychology, Crime, and Law, 10*, 413–427.

Hare, R. D. (1991). *The Revised Psychopathy Checklist.* Toronto, ON: Multi-Health Systems.

Hare, R. D. (2003). *The Psychopathy Checklist* (2nd ed.). Toronto, ON: Multi-Health Systems.

Harris, G. T., Rice, M. E. & Camilleri, J. A. (2004) Applying a forensic actuarial assessment (the Violence Risk Appraisal Guide) to nonforensic patients. *Journal of Interpersonal Violence, 19*, 1063–1074..

*Heckert, D. A., & Gondolf, E. W. (2000). The effect of perceptions of sanctions on batterer program outcomes. *Journal of Research in Crime and Delinquency, 37*, 369–391.

Heckert, D. A., & Gondolf, E. W. (2004). Battered women's perceptions of risk versus risk factors and instruments in predicting repeat reassault. *Journal of Interpersonal Violence, 19*, 778–800.

Heyman, R. E., O'Leary, K. D., & Jouriles, E. N. (1995). Alcohol and aggressive personality styles: Potentiators of serious physical aggression against wives? *Journal of Family Psychology, 9*, 44–57.

Hilton, N. Z. (1989). One in ten: The struggle and disempowerment of the battered women's movement. *Canadian Journal of Family Law, 7*, 313–336.

Hilton, N. Z., & Harris, G. T. (2005). The prediction of wife assault: A critical review and implications for policy and practice. *Trauma, Violence, & Abuse, 6*, 3–23.

*Hilton, N. Z., & Harris, G. T. (2007). *Replication of the ODARA: The definition of nonrecidivism affects apparent prediction accuracy*. Manuscript submitted for publication.

Hilton, N. Z., & Harris, G. T. (in press). Criminal justice responses to partner violence: History, evaluation, and lessons from interventions for criminal conduct. In J. Lutzker & D. Whitaker (Eds.), *Preventing partner violence: Foundations, intervention, issues*. Washington, DC: American Psychological Association.

Hilton, N. Z., Harris, G. T., Rawson, K., & Beach, C. A. (2005). Communicating violence risk information to forensic decision makers. *Criminal Justice and Behavior, 32*, 97–116.

*Hilton, N. Z., Harris, G. T., & Rice, M. E. (2001). Predicting violence by serious wife assaulters. *Journal of Interpersonal Violence, 16*, 408–423.

Hilton, N. Z., Harris, G. T., & Rice, M. E. (2006). Sixty-six years of research on clinical versus actuarial prediction of violence. *The Counseling Psychologist, 34*, 400–409.

Hilton, N. Z., Harris, G. T., & Rice, M. E. (in press). *The decision to arrest for wife assault and the effect on recidivism. Criminal Justice and Behavior.*

*Hilton, N. Z., Harris, G. T., Rice, M. E., Houghton, R. E., & Eke, A. W. (in press). An indepth risk assessment for wife assault recidivism: General antisociality and domain-specific prediction and explanation. *Law and Human Behavior.*

Hilton, N. Z., Harris, G. T., Rice, M. E., Lang, C., Cormier, C. A., & Lines, K. J. (2004). A brief actuarial assessment for the prediction of wife assault recidivism: The Ontario Domestic Assault Risk Assessment. *Psychological Assessment, 16*, 267-275.

Hilton, N. Z., & Simmons, J. L. (2001). The influence of actuarial risk assessment and clinical judgments in tribunal decisions about mentally disordered offenders. *Law and Human Behavior, 4*, 391–406.

Hines, D. A., & Saudino, K. J. (2002). Intergenerational transmission of intimate partner violence: A behavioral genetic perspective. *Trauma, Violence, & Abuse, 3*, 210–225.

Hines, D. A., & Saudino, K. J. (2004). Genetic and environmental influences on intimate partner aggression: A preliminary study. *Violence and Victims, 19*, 701–718.

Holtzworth-Munroe, A., Bates, L., Smutzler, N., & Sandin, E. (1997). A brief review of the research on husband violence. *Aggression and Violent Behavior, 2*, 65–99.

Huss, M. T., Covell, C. N. & Langhinrichsen-Rohling, J. (2006). Clinical implications for the assessment and treatment of antisocial and psychopathic domestic violence perpetrators. *Journal of Aggression, Maltreatment, & Trauma, 13*, 58–86.

Huss, M. T., & Langhinrichsen-Rohling, J. (2000). Identification of the psychopathic batterer: The clinical, legal, and policy implications. *Aggression and Violent Behavior, 5*, 403–442.

Jacobson, N. S., Gottman, J. M., Gortner, E., Berns, W., & Shortt, J. W. (1996). Psychological factors in the longitudinal course of battering: When do the couples split up? When does the abuse decrease? *Violence and Victims, 11*, 371–392.

Jasinski, J. L. (2001). Physical violence among Anglo, African American, and Hispanic couples: Ethnic differences in persistence and cessation. *Violence and Victims, 16*, 479–490.

*Kropp, P. R., & Hart, S. D. (2000). The Spousal Assault Risk Assessment (SARA) Guide: Reliability and validity in adult male offenders. *Law and Human Behavior, 24*, 101–118.

Kropp, P. R., Hart, S. D., Webster, C. D., & Eaves, D. (1999). *Spousal Assault Risk Assessment Guide (SARA)*. Toronto, ON: Multi-Health Systems Inc.

Lalumière, M. L., Harris, G. T., Quinsey, V. L., & Rice, M. E., (2005). The causes of rape: *Understanding individual differences in the male propensity for sexual aggression*. Washington, DC: American Psychological Association.

Landau, T. C. (2000). Women's experiences with mandatory charging for wife assault in Ontario, Canada: A case against the prosecution. *International Review of Victimology, 7*, 141–157.

Leonard, K. E., & Roberts, L. J. (1998). The effects of alcohol on the marital interactions of aggressive and nonaggressive husbands and their wives. *Journal of Abnormal Psychology, 107*, 602–615.

Leonard, K. E., & Senchak, M. (1996). Prospective prediction of husband marital aggression within newlywed couples. *Journal of Abnormal Psychology, 105*, 369–380.

Levinson, D. (1989). Family violence in cross-cultural perspective. Newbury Park, CA: Sage.

Logan, T. K., Walker, R., Jordan, C. E., & Leukefeld, C. G. (2006). *Women and victimization*. Washington, DC: American Psychological Association.

Marshall, A. D., & Holtzworth-Munroe, A. (2002). Varying forms of husband sexual aggression: Predictors and subgroup differences. *Journal of Family Psychology, 16*, 286–296.

Martin, M. E. (1997). Double your trouble: Dual arrest in family violence. *Journal of Family Violence, 12*, 139-157.

McBurnett, K., Kerckhoff, C., Capasso, L., Pfiffner, L. J., Rathouz, P. J., & Harris, S. M. (2001). Antisocial personality, substance abuse, and exposure to parental violence in males referred for domestic violence. *Violence and Victims, 16*, 491–506.

Monson, C. M., & Langhinrichsen-Rohling, J. (1998). Sexual and nonsexual marital aggression: Legal considerations, epidemiology, and an integrated typology of perpetrators. *Aggression and Violent Behavior, 3*, 369–389.

Murphy, C. M., O'Farrell, T. J., Fals-Stewart, W., & Feehan, M. (2001). Correlates of intimate partner violence among male alcoholic patients. *Journal of Consulting and Clinical Psychology, 69*, 528–540.

O'Leary, K. D., Barling, J., Arias, I., Rosenbaum, A., Malone, A., Malone, J., et al. (1989). Prevalence and stability of physical aggression between spouses: A longitudinal analysis. *Journal of Consulting and Clinical Psychology, 57*, 263–268.

O'Leary, K. D., & Curley, A. D. (1986). Assertion and family violence: Correlates of spouse abuse. *Journal of Marital and Family Therapy, 12*, 281–289.

O'Leary, K. D., Malone, J., & Tyree, A. (1994). Physical aggression in early marriage: Prerelationship and relationship effects. *Journal of Consulting and Clinical Psychology, 62*, 594–602.

Quigley, B. M., & Leonard, K. E. (1996). Desistance of husband aggression in the early years of marriage. *Violence and Victims, 11*, 355–370.

Quinsey, V. L., Harris, G. T., Rice, M. E., & Cormier, C. A. (2006). *Violent offenders: Appraising and managing risk* (2nd ed.). Washington, DC: American Psychological Association.

Ramirez, I. L. (2005). Criminal history and assaults on intimate partners by Mexican American and Non-Mexican White college students. *Journal of Interpersonal Violence, 20,* 1628-1647.

Rennison, C. M., & Welchans, S. (2000). Intimate partner violence. *Bureau of Justice Statistics Special Report,* 1–11.

Rice, M. E., & Harris, G. T. (1995). Violent recidivism: Assessing predictive validity. *Journal of Consulting and Clinical Psychology, 63*, 737–748.

Rice, M. E., & Harris, G. T. (2003). What we know and don't know about treating sex offenders. In B. J. Winick and J. Q. LaFond (Eds.), *Protecting society from sexually dangerous offenders: Law, justice and therapy* (pp. 101–117). Washington, DC: American Psychological Association.

Rice, M. E., & Harris, G. T. (2005). Comparing effect sizes in follow-up studies: ROC, Cohen's d and r. *Law and Human Behavior, 29*, 615–620.

Roehl, J., & Guertin, K. (2000). Intimate partner violence: The current use of risk assessments in sentencing offenders. *The Justice System Journal, 21*, 171–198.

Rooney, J., & Hanson, R. K. (2001). Predicting attrition from treatment programs for abusive men. *Journal of Family Violence, 16*, 131–149.

Saunders, D. G. (1995). Prediction of wife assault. In J. C. Campbell (Ed.), *Assessing dangerousness: Violence by sexual offenders, batterers, and child abusers* (pp. 68–95). Thousand Oaks, CA: Sage.

Seto, M. C., & Barbaree, H. E. (1999). Psychopathy, treatment behavior, and sex offender recidivism. *Journal of Interpersonal Violence,14,* 1235–1248.

Shackelford, T. K., Buss, D. M., & Peters, J. (2000). Wife killing: Risk to women as a function of age. *Violence and Victims, 15*, 273–282.

Shackelford, T. K., Buss, D. M., & Weekes-Shackelford, V. A. (2003). Wife killings committed in the context of a lovers triangle. *Basic and Applied Social Psychology, 25*, 137–143.

Sharps, P. W., Campbell, J., Campbell, D., Foy, G., & Webster, D. (2001). The role of alcohol use in intimate partner femicide. *American Journal on Addictions, 10*, 122–136.

Shepard, M. F., Falk, D. R., & Elliott, B. A. (2002). Enhancing coordinated community responses to reduce recidivism in cases of domestic violence. *Journal of Interpersonal Violence, 17*, 551–569.

Sherman, L. W. & Berk, R. A. (1984). The specific deterrent effects of arrest for domestic assault. *American Sociological Review, 49,* 261-272.

Skuja, K., & Halford, W. K. (2004). Repeating the errors of our parents? *Journal of Interpersonal Violence, 19,* 623–638.

Stark, E., & Flitcraft, A. (1996). *Women at risk.* Thousand Oaks, CA: Sage.

Straus, M. A. (1983). Ordinary violence, child abuse, and wife-beating. In D. Finkelhor, R. J. Gelles, G. T. Hotaling, & M. A. Straus (Eds.), *The dark side of families* (pp. 213–234). Beverly Hills, CA: Sage.

Straus, M. A., & Ramirez, I. L. (2004). Criminal history and assault of dating partners: The role of type of prior crime, age of onset, and gender. *Violence and Victims, 19,* 413–434.

Thompson, M. P., & Kingree, J. B. (2006). The roles of victim and perpetrator alcohol use in intimate partner violence. *Journal of Interpersonal Violence, 21,* 163–177.

Torres, S., Campbell, J., Campbell, D. W., Ryan, J., King, C., Price, P., et al. (2000). Abuse during and before pregnancy: Prevalence and cultural correlates. *Violence and Victims, 15,* 303–321.

Tutty, L. M., Bidgood, B. A., Rothery, M. A., & Bidgood, P. (2001). An evaluation of men's batterer treatment groups. *Research on Social Work Practice, 11,* 645–670.

*Weisz, A. N., Tolman, R. M., & Saunders, D. G. (2000). Assessing the risk of severe domestic violence: The importance of survivors' predictions. *Journal of Interpersonal Violence, 15,* 75–90.

Williams, K. R., & Grant, S. R. (2006). Empirically examining the risk of intimate partner violence: The Revised Domestic Violence screening Instrument (DVSI R). *Public Health Reports, 121,* 400–408

*Williams, K. R., & Houghton, A. B. (2004). Assessing the risk of domestic violence reoffending: A validation study. *Law and Human Behavior, 28,* 437–455.

Wilson, M., & Daly, M. (1998). Lethal and nonlethal violence against wives and the evolutionary psychology of male sexual proprietariness. In R. E. Dobash & R. P. Dobash (Eds.), *Rethinking violence against women* (pp. 199–249). Thousand Oaks, CA: Sage.

CHAPTER 7

Risk Factors for Femicide-Suicide in Abusive Relationships: Results From a Multisite Case Control Study*

Jane Koziol-McLain, Daniel Webster,
Judith McFarlane, Carolyn Rebecca Block,
Yvonne Ulrich, Nancy Glass, and
Jacquelyn C. Campbell

It is estimated that 1,000 to 1,500 homicide-suicide deaths occur annually in the United States (Brock, 2002; Marzuk, Tardiff, & Hirsch, 1992). Our understanding of the epidemiology of homicide followed by suicide, however, is hampered by the lack of a national surveillance system (Hannah, Turf, & Fierro, 1998; Malphurs & Cohen, 2002; Paulozzi, Mercy, Frazier, & Annest, 2004). Databases relied upon for homicide and suicide rates, such as the Supplemental Homicide Report and National Vital Statistics System, are unable to link homicide to suicide events. The CDC National Violent Death Reporting System (NVDRS) is purported to correct this surveillance inadequacy (Paulozzi et al., 2004), but the first report from the NVDRS did not include homicide-suicide data (National Center for Injury Prevention and Control CDC, 2005). Until linked data are available, researchers have had to rely on police and medical examiner record review and follow-up

*This chapter was previously published in *Violence and Victims* (Springer Publishing Company), 2006, Vol. 21, No. 1, pp. 3–21.

interviews (a reasonable task only for small studies) or search newspaper clippings for case identification (Brock, 2002; Cohen, Llorente, & Eisdorfer, 1998; Lund & Smorodinsky, 2001; Malphurs & Cohen, 2002). Despite these methodologic limitations, a growing body of international literature confirms that homicide-suicide is patterned. Homicide is more likely to be followed by suicide when there is a close bond between the victim and perpetrator, with intimate partners—followed by children—most commonly killed, and following male perpetrators killing female partners (Aderibigbe, 1997; Allen, 1983; Barraclough & Harris, 2002; Brock, 2002; Buteau, Lesage, & Kiely, 1993; Campanelli & Gilson, 2002; Chan, Beh, & Broadburst, 2004; Currens et al., 1991; Gillespie, Hearn, & Silverman, 1998; Hannah et al., 1998; Lecomte & Fornes, 1998; Malphurs & Cohen, 2002; Milroy, Dratsas, & Ranson, 1997; Palermo et al., 1997; Polk, 1994; Rosenbaum, 1990; Stack, 1997; Websdale, 1999; Wolfgang, 1958). For example, a review of firearm homicides in Kentucky (1998–2000) found that when an intimate partner was killed (46), 70% involved a male killing his partner followed by killing himself (Walsh & Hemenway, 2005), confirming an earlier Kentucky homicide review (Currens et al., 1991). Across studies, approximately 25% of intimate partner femicides (homicide of women) in the United States, Australia, Canada, and Sweden are followed by suicide, compared to less than 5% of nonintimate killings (Belfrage & Rying, 2004; Cooper & Eaves, 1996; Dawson & Gartner, 1998; Easteal, 1993; Easteal, 1994; Johnson & Hotton, 2003; Lund & Smorodinsky, 2001; Morton, Runyan, Moracco, & Butts, 1998; Rosenbaum, 1990).

One theoretical explanation for femicide-suicide is that the perpetrator becomes remorseful after killing his source of nurturance and commits suicide (Stack, 1997; Wolfgang, 1958). This explanation, however, is challenged by the premeditated nature of the majority of femicide-suicides (Cooper & Eaves, 1996; Dawson & Gartner, 1998; Dawson, 2005; Marzuk et al., 1992) and the immediacy between the two acts (Cooper & Eaves, 1996). Several homicide-suicide researchers have developed and used homicide-suicide typologies (Belfrage & Rying, 2004; Campanelli & Gilson, 2002; Dawson, 2005; Felthous & Hempel, 1995; Hannah et al., 1998; Lecomte & Fornes, 1998; Malphurs & Cohen, 2002; Marzuk et al., 1992; Morton et al., 1998), though many of these fail to take into account the gendered nature of homicide-suicides and the history of abuse within relationships. Several authors include mercy killing, when failing health prevents caregiving, as a homicide-suicide trigger among older adults (Allen, 1983; Easteal, 1993; Malphurs & Cohen, 2002; Marzuk et al., 1992). However, Malphurs and Cohen (2005) recently found perpetrator caregiving strain and domestic violence differentiated older adult homicide-suicide from older adult homicide; Dawson (2005), examining homicide-suicides in Ontario, reported that in 12 of 14 cases attributed to mercy killing there was no indication that the victim had been involved in the decision that ended her life. Mental illness, most notably depression, is another contributory factor cited in the literature. However, the proportion of perpetrators reported to have been depressed varies widely across studies, from between 15% and 86% (Bourget, Gagne, & Moamai, 2000; Buteau et al., 1993; Campanelli & Gilson, 2002; Cohen et al., 1998; Cooper & Eaves, 1996; Lecomte & Fornes, 1998; Malphurs, Eisdorfer, & Cohen, 2001; Morton et al., 1998; Rosenbaum, 1990). The majority of these studies did not standardize data concerning perpetrator depression or suicidality, and psychological reports were rarely available (Rosenbaum, 1990).

A more recent theoretical explanation for femicide-suicide relates to male proprietariness, a pathological possessiveness that deals with power and control (Campanelli & Gilson, 2002; Cooper & Eaves, 1996; Lecomte & Fornes, 1998; Polk, 1994; Rosenbaum, 1990; Wilson & Daly, 1993a). That femicide-suicides typically occur following estrangement and are planned acts support this explanation. Yet this explanation is incomplete, combining proprietariness and perpetrator personality disorder(s) may account for his placing such high stakes on his relationship (and possessiveness) with his partner (Rosenbaum, 1990). Interestingly, the constant across the literature is the perpetrator statement, "If I can't have you nobody can"; this statement, however, is also noted in femicide without suicide. Most authors acknowledge the explanations for femicide-suicide, where no witnesses survive, is difficult to prove and most likely involves, as Easteal (Hillbrand, 2002) says, "a mosaic" of causes.

Despite the various explanations for femicide-suicide, it commonly occurs following an estrangement (Bourget et al., 2000; Buteau et al., 1993; Cooper & Eaves, 1996; Dawson, 2005; Johnson & Hotton, 2003; Lecomte & Fornes, 1998; Morton et al., 1998; Palermo et al., 1997; Rosenbaum, 1990; Wilson & Daly, 1993b); in relationships where the male perpetrator has physically battered his partner over time (Campanelli & Gilson, 2002; Lecomte & Fornes, 1998; Morton et al., 1998; Rosenbaum, 1990); and in the United States, Australia, Canada, and France, if a firearm was used (Aderibigbe, 1997; Allen, 1983; Bourget et al., 2000; Campbell et al., 2003; Cooper & Eaves, 1996; Dawson, 2005; Easteal, 1994; Gillespie et al., 1998; Hannah et al., 1998; Lund & Smorodinsky, 2001; Malphurs & Cohen, 2002; Milroy et al., 1997; Morton et al., 1998; Palermo et al., 1997). However, these three characteristics are common among all intimate partner femicides. In reviewing the literature, all previous studies examined femicide-suicide cases alone, or compared femicide-suicide cases to femicide (without suicide) cases. Yet in both femicide and femicide-suicide cases, the outcome is death. Assessments regarding suicide and homicide risk are generally known, yet little is known about the dynamic relationship between suicide and homicide risk (Hillbrand, 2002).

In this study we wanted to learn whether there are unique femicide-suicide risk factors that should be assessed at a point of contact with either partner violence victims or perpetrators in order to intervene and prevent this lethal tragedy. Therefore, we conducted an analysis examining the relative risk factors for intimate partner femicide-suicide among women in violent relationships with the aim to inform prevention and intervention efforts. The analysis comes from a multisite study of risk factors for intimate partner femicide (Campbell et al., 2003).

METHOD

Femicide risk was studied in a case control study across 11 U.S. cities: New York, NY; Baltimore, MD; Tampa, FL; Chicago, IL; Kansas City, MO; Kansas City, KS; Wichita, KS; Houston, TX; Los Angeles, CA; Portland, OR; and Seattle, WA (Campbell et al., 2003). Consecutive femicide cases 1994 through 2000 were identified through police and medical examiner records and subsequently reviewed to determine whether the perpetrator was a current or former intimate partner of the victim. Of 545 identified femicide cases, risk data were available (successful interview of victim proxy) for 310. Controls ($n = 356$) were identified via a phone survey using random digit dialing within the same cities in which cases were identified and were eligible if they were female, 18 to 50 years of age, and had been physically abused by a current or former intimate partner within the past 2 years. Among 4,746 women who met age and relationship criteria, 3,637 (77%) agreed to participate and 356 (9.8%) met physical abuse criteria.

A detailed questionnaire was developed that examined the demographics of the victim and perpetrator (intimate or ex-intimate partner), characteristics of the relationship and intimate partner violence, and characteristics of the "worst incident" for controls and the femicide event for the cases. While some questions were developed by the research team, the majority were from established instruments such as the Danger Assessment (Campbell, 1995). The questionnaire was administered in either English or Spanish (following translation and back-translation). For controls, women themselves answered the questionnaire. For women who were killed, proxy informants were interviewed. Proxy informants were most often sisters, mothers, or girlfriends of the killed women. The study protocol received ethical approval by Institutional Review Boards in each of the participating cities; consent was obtained from all participants (controls and proxy informants) following full disclosure of study benefits and risks. Police files and medical examiner reports were also examined for femicide cases. Variables are more thoroughly described in a previous publication (Campbell et al., 2003; National Center for Injury Prevention and Control CDC, 2005). In this analysis we examined the femicide cases that were followed by suicide and compared risk factors among femicide-suicide cases and controls.

Femicide-Suicide Cases

Femicide-suicide cases were selected for analysis from among all femicide cases based on control criteria, that is, 18 to 50 years of age and prior partner abuse. Among the 310 femicide cases, 100 (32%) were followed by suicide (Figure 7.1). In 72% of femicide-suicide cases there was evidence of a history of physical abuse by the perpetrator in the year prior to the killing, this compares to 77% among femicide without suicide cases and 9.8% among the population-based sample of women who agreed to be interviewed for the control group. Excluding cases outside the age range and without a history of abuse, 67 femicide-suicide cases were selected for case-control analysis of femicide-suicide risk factors.

Data Analysis

First, bivariate analyses were done comparing femicide-suicide characteristics to controls. Characteristics of femicide without suicide are also presented and will be referred to in the discussion to elucidate factors that are unique to femicide-suicide. Then, logistic regression was used to estimate the independent association between the hypothesized risk factors and the risk of femicide-suicide. Sequentially added blocks of explanatory variables ordered along a continuum moving closer to the violent event were entered into the regression models. This conceptualization was helpful in organizing the many variables and allowed us to examine whether some risk factors (e.g., patterns of preincident physical abuse, incident-level weapon use) mediate the effects of more distal risk factors (e.g., gun ownership) in the progression from earlier in the intimate relationship to the femicide-suicide event. Dichotomous threatening and abusive behavior variables that were unknown by victims' proxies were conservatively set to "no" for the regression analysis. Variables not significantly associated with femicide-suicide risk ($p > .05$) were dropped from subsequent models. Annual household income was missing for 28% of the abused women, and therefore not entered into the model.

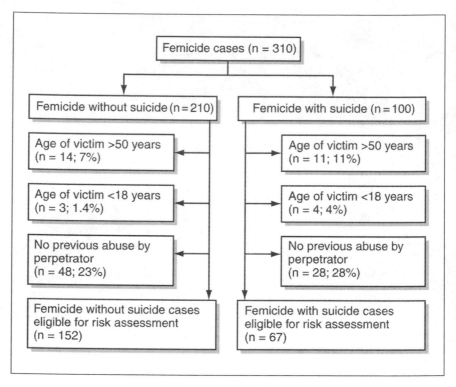

FIGURE 7. 1. Femicide case selection with and without suicide.

Note. Age of victim and previous partner abuse are not mutually exclusive, therefore numbers do not sum.

Logistic regression was used to estimate adjusted odds ratios (aOR). It is important to note that substantial changes in coefficients from one model to the next may indicate mediation, particularly when mediation is theoretically plausible. The small sample size, however, prohibited examination of inter-actions. The Hosmer and Lemeshow goodness-of-fit test probabilities were nonsignificant across all the models. While there are differences in calculating logistic regression model variance compared to ordinary least squares (OLS) multiple regression, the Nagelkerke pseudo R^2 measure is reported to facilitate examination of explained variance across the models (SPSS, 2001).

RESULTS

Sociodemographics

Femicide-suicide partners (the perpetrators), compared to abused control male partners, were slightly older (mean age 35 versus 31 years), had left school earlier (8% versus 26% having graduated college) and were more often unemployed not seeking a job (28% versus. 13%; Table 7.1). Femicide-suicide abused women (the victims), compared to abused control women, had left school earlier (14% versus 28% college graduate), and were less likely to have an annual household income below $10, 000 (8% versus 22%), though income information was often missing. There were no differences in victim's employment or in victim or perpetrator race and ethnicity.

General Violence

Femicide-suicide partners, compared to abused control partners, were more likely to have made suicide threats (51% versus 20%), have an alcohol problem (52% versus 32%), and used illicit drugs (50% versus 31%; Table 7.1). Femicide-suicide abused women, compared to abused control women, were more likely to have poor mental health (21% versus 11%), yet fewer suicide threats (0% versus 10%). The difference in proportions for access to guns was striking: 81% of femicide-suicide cases reported gun access versus 25% among controls. There were trivial differences in women's alcohol and drug use between the two groups.

Relationship

Femicide-suicide cases were more likely to involve husbands (52% versus 29%) and to occur following an estrangement (Table 7.2). Fifty-two percent of the femicide-suicide cases involved a couple that was estranged (versus 36%), although their marital status may still be "married." Consistent with estrangement, more femicide-suicide cases lived together within the past year but not at the time of the worst incident (39% versus 12%). In addition, the age difference between victims and perpetrators was greater for femicide-suicides than for the controls (3.1 versus 1.1 years, male partners being older). Having one or more child living in the household who was not fathered by the perpetrator was more common in femicide-suicide households (45% versus 17%).

Abuse Dynamics

Both high control (69% versus 26%) and name calling (75% versus 48%) were more common among femicide-suicide cases than among controls.

Threatening Behaviors

All measures of threatening behaviors differentiated femicide-suicide from controls (Table 7.2). These included threat(s) to kill the woman (78% versus 16%), threat(s) to kill the family (33% versus 8%), threat(s) with a weapon

TABLE 7.1 Sociodemographic and General Violence Characteristics of Abused Women and Their Abusive Partners by Group[a]

	Abused			Abusive Partners		
	Controls (n = 356) n (%)	Femicide W/ Suicide (n = 67) n (%)	Femicide W/O Suicide (n = 152) n (%)	Controls (n = 356) n (%)	Femicide W/ Suicide (n = 67) n (%)	Femicide W/O Suicide (n = 152) n (%)
Sociodemographics						
Age (mean age years ± SD)	30.0 ± 8.5	31.5 ± 8.2	31.2 ± 7.5	31.1 ± 9.1	34.6 ± 8.4	34.0 ± 8.9
Don't know/refused/missing	0	0	0	4	8	13
		p = .17	*p* = .113		*p* = .005	*p* < .01
Race/ethnicity						
Black/African American	78 (22.2)	22 (32.8)	81 (53.3)	90 (25.4)	24 (35.8)	82 (54.3)
White	160 (45.5)	21 (31.3)	32 (21.1)	156 (43.9)	19 (28.4)	30 (19.9)
Latino/Hispanic	84 (23.9)	20 (29.9)	33 (21.7)	83 (23.4)	20 (29.9)	38 (25.2)
Other	30 (8.5)	4 (6.0)	6 (3.9)	26 (7.3)	4 (6.0)	1 (0.7)
Don't know/refused/missing	4	0	0	1	0	0
		p = .09	*p* < .01		*p* = .09	*p* < .01
Education						
< high school	63 (17.8)	19 (29.2)	51 (34.5)	96 (28.3)	19 (37.3)	51 (55.4)
High school diploma/GED	80 (22.7)	12 (18.5)	47 (31.8)	97 (28.6)	18 (35.3)	29 (31.5)
Some college/trade school	112 (31.7)	25 (38.5)	43 (29.1)	59 (17.4)	10 (19.6)	7 (7.6)
College/trade school graduate	98 (27.8)	9 (13.8)	7 (4.7)	87 (25.7)	4 (7.8)	5 (5.4)
Don't know/refused/missing	3	2	4	17	16	60
		p = .03	*p* < .01		*p* = .045	*p* < .01
Employment						
Full-time	185 (52.0)	44 (65.7)	70 (46.1)	236 (67.6)	37 (57.8)	47 (32.0)
Part-time	74 (20.8)	10 (14.9)	21 (13.8)	42 (12.0)	6 (9.4)	14 (9.5)
Unemployed, seeking job	43 (12.1)	2 (3.0)	10 (6.6)	25 (7.2)	3 (4.7)	10 (6.8)

Unemployed, not seeking job	54 (15.2)	11 (16.4)	51 (33.6)	46 (13.2)	18 (28.1)	76 (51.7)
Don't know/refused/missing	0	0	0	7	3	5
		p = .06	**p < .01**		**p = .02**	**p < .01**
Income (annual household)						
< $10,000	71 (22.1)	4 (8.3)	21 (24.7)			
$10,000–$19,999	51 (15.9)	7 (14.6)	25 (29.4)			
$20,000–$29,999	48 (14.9)	7 (14.6)	13 (15.3)			
$30,000–$39,000	41 (12.8)	13 (27.1)	16 (18.8)			
>= $40,000	110 (34.3)	17 (35.4)	10 (11.8)			
Don't know/refused/missing	35	19	67			
		p = .044	**p < .01**			
General violence indicators						
Physical health						
Excellent/good	286 (81.9)	60 (89.6)	111 (73.0)	275 (79.0)	49 (79.0)	112 (81.2)
Fair	48 (13.8)	3 (4.5)	27 (17.8)	53 (15.2)	10 (16.1)	19 (13.8)
Poor	15 (4.3)	4 (6.0)	14 (9.2)	20 (5.7)	3 (4.8)	7 (5.1)
Don't know/refused/missing	0	0	0	5	5	15
		p = .09	p = .04		p = .95	p = .87
Mental health						
Excellent/good	238 (67.6)	47 (70.1)	103 (68.2)	171 (48.7)	21 (34.4)	63 (49.6)
Fair	75 (21.3)	6 (9.0)	26 (17.2)	93 (26.5)	17 (27.9)	28 (22.0)
Poor	39 (11.1)	14 (20.9)	22 (14.6)	87 (24.8)	23 (37.7)	36 (28.3)
Don't know/refused/missing	0	0	1	6	6	25
		p = .01	p = .38		p = .06	p = .55
Suicide threats						
Yes	37 (10.4)	0	12 (8.1)	70 (19.9)	28 (50.9)	17 (13.6)
No	319 (89.6)	65 (100)	136 (91.9)	282 (80.1)	27 (49.1)	108 (86.4)
Don't know/refused/missing	2	2	5	12	12	27
		p < .01	p = .43		**p < .01**	p = .12
Alcohol problem						
Yes	28 (7.9)	3 (5.4)	32 (24.4)	112 (31.5)	32 (51.6)	72 (51.8)

(Continued)

TABLE 7.1 Sociodemographic and General Violence Characteristics of Abused Women and Their Abusive Partners by Group[a] (Continued)

	Abused			Abusive Partners		
	Controls (n = 356) n (%)	Femicide W/ Suicide (n = 67) n (%)	Femicide W/O Suicide (n = 152) n (%)	Controls (n = 356) n (%)	Femicide W/ Suicide (n = 67) n (%)	Femicide W/O Suicide (n = 152) n (%)
No	328 (92.1)	53 (94.6)	99 (75.6)	244 (68.5)	30 (48.4)	67 (48.2)
Don't know/refused/missing		11	21		5	13
		$p = .51$	$p < .01$		$p < .01$	$p < .01$
General violence indicators						
Illicit drug use						
Yes	51 (14.4)	6 (10.0)	41 (31.8)	108 (31.3)	29 (50.0)	93 (72.1)
No	304 (85.6)	54 (90.0)	88 (68.2)	237 (68.7)	29 (50.0)	36 (27.9)
Don't know/refused/missing	1	7	23	11	9	23
		$p = .36$	$p < .01$		$p < .01$	$p < .01$
Access to guns[b]						
Yes	18 (5.1)	1 (1.6)	9 (6.5)	90 (25.3)	54 (80.6)	89 (58.6)
No	336 (94.9)	60 (98.4)	130 (93.5)	266 (74.7)	13 (19.4)	63 (41.4)
Don't know/refused/missing	2	6	13	0	0	0
		$p = .23$	$p = .54$		$p < .01$	$p < .01$
Arrest for violent crime						
Yes				42 (12.2)	11 (18.3)	32 (23.4)
No				302 (87.8)	49 (81.7)	105 (76.6)
Don't know/refused/missing				12	7	15
					$p = .19$	$p < .01$

[a] p values are for comparisons between femicide group (with or without suicide) and controls based on chi-square tests for categorical variables and independent t tests for continuous variables; p values less than .05 are in boldface.
[b] Gun access for abused women based on living separate from their partner and reporting a gun in the home; gun access for partner based on living together and reporting a gun in the home.

TABLE 7.2   Relationship Dynamics, Threatening Behavior, and Abuse Characteristics

	Controls (n = 356) n (%)	Femicide W/ Suicide (n = 67) n (%)	Femicide W/O Suicide (n = 152) n (%)
Relationship characteristics			
Age difference			
(partner minus abused woman;	1.1 ± 5.7	3.1 ± 5.8	2.8 ± 6.6
mean ± SD)		8	13
		p = .01	p = .01
Relationship			
Husband	103 (29.2)	34 (51.5)	50 (33.1)
Boyfriend	88 (24.9)	12 (18.2)	53 (35.1)
Ex-husband	39 (11.0)	8 (12.1)	12 (7.9)
Ex-boyfriend	123 (34.8)	12 (18.2)	36 (23.8)
Don't know/refused/missing	3	1	1
		p = .002	p = .023
Separated			
Yes	126 (36.2)	31 (52.5)	70 (56.9)
No	222 (63.8)	28 (47.5)	53 (43.1)
Don't know/refused/missing	8	8	29
		p = .02	p < .01
Cohabitation (living together)			
Yes	178 (50.0)	28 (49.1)	52 (42.6)
In the past year, but not currently	44 (12.4)	22 (38.6)	46 (37.7)
Not in the past year	12 (3.4)	1 (1.8)	10 (8.2)
Never	122 (34.3)	6 (10.5)	14 (11.5)
Don't know/refused/missing	0	10	30
		p < .01	p < .01
Biological child(ren) of abused and			
partner living in the household			
Yes	102 (28.7)	20 (33.9)	52 (38.5)
No	254 (71.3)	39 (66.1)	83 (61.5)
Don't know/refused/missing	0	8	17
		p = .41	p = .038
Biological child(ren) of abused,			
and not of partner living in			
the household			
Yes	61 (17.1)	29 (44.6)	52 (35.6)
No	295 (82.9)	36 (55.4)	94 (64.4)
Don't know/refused/missing	0	2	6
		p < .01	p < .01
Relationship abuse dynamics			
Partner controlling behaviors			
(score > 3)			
Yes	91 (25.6)	46 (68.7)	98 (64.5)

(Continued)

TABLE 7.2   Relationship Dynamics, Threatening Behavior, and Abuse Characteristics (*Continued*)

	Controls (n = 356) n (%)	Femicide W/ Suicide (n = 67) n (%)	Femicide W/O Suicide (n = 152) n (%)
No	265 (74.4)	21 (31.3)	54 (35.5)
Don't know/refused/missing	0	0	0
		p < .01	*p* < .01
Partner called her names to put her down			
Yes	171 (48.0)	47 (74.6)	103 (79.2)
No	185 (52.0)	16 (25.4)	27 (20.8)
Don't know/refused/missing	0	4	22
		p < .01	*p* < .01
Threatening behaviors			
Partner violent outside home			
Yes	124 (36.5)	29 (51.8)	73 (57.9)
No	216 (63.5)	27 (48.2)	53 (42.1)
Don't know/refused/missing	16	11	26
		p = .03	*p* < .01
Partner threatened to kill woman			
Yes	56 (15.8)	47 (78.3)	94 (71.2)
No	299 (84.2)	13 (21.7)	38 (28.8)
Don't know/refused/missing	1	7	20
		p < .01	*p* < .01
Partner threatened to kill family			
Yes	28 (7.9)	22 (33.3)	50 (34.2)
No	328 (92.1)	44 (66.7)	96 (65.8)
Don't know/refused/missing	0	1	6
		p < .01	*p* < .01
Partner threatened woman with a weapon			
Yes	18 (5.1)	35 (55.6)	75 (55.6)
No	338 (94.9)	28 (44.4)	60 (44.4)
Don't know/refused/missing	0	4	17
		p < .01	*p* < .01
Partner threatened to take children			
Yes	39 (11.3)	13 (19.7)	24 (17.5)
No	307 (88.7)	53 (80.3)	113 (82.5)
Don't know/refused/missing	10	1	15
		p < .01	*p* < .01
Stalking behavior (score > 3)			
Yes	23 (6.5)	16 (23.9)	31 (20.4)

(Continued)

TABLE 7.2 *(Continued)*

	Controls (n = 356) n (%)	Femicide W/ Suicide (n = 67) n (%)	Femicide W/O Suicide (n = 152) n (%)
No	333 (93.5)	51 (76.1)	121 (79.6)
Don't know/refused/missing	0	0	0
		p < .01	p < .01
Characteristics of physical violence			
Increase in frequency			
Yes	91 (25.9)	32 (59.3)	76 (59.8)
No	260 (74.1)	22 (40.7)	51 (40.2)
Don't know/refused/missing	5	13	25
		p < .01	p < .01
Increase in severity			
Yes	72 (20.5)	31 (56.4)	74 (57.4)
No	279 (79.5)	24 (43.6)	55 (42.6)
Don't know/refused/missing	5	12	23
		p < .01	p < .01
Partner tried to choke (strangle) woman			
Yes	41 (11.5)	26 (52.0)	57 (58.2)
No	314 (88.5)	24 (48.0)	41 (41.8)
Don't know/refused/missing	1	17	54
		p < .01	p < .01
Forced sex			
Yes	53 (14.9)	29 (56.9)	55 (57.3)
No	302 (85.1)	22 (43.1)	41 (42.7)
Don't know/refused/missing	1	16	56
		p < .01	p < .01
Abused during pregnancy (ever)			
Yes	30 (8.4)	8 (13.8)	40 (30.5)
No or never been pregnant	326 (91.6)	50 (86.2)	91 (69.5)
Don't know/refused/missing	0	9	21
		p = .19	p < .01
Partner prior arrest for domestic violence			
Yes	52 (15.1%)	14 (23.7)	36 (26.5)
No	292 (84.9%)	45 (76.3)	100 (73.5)
Don't know/refused/missing	12	8	16
		p = .09	p < .01
Incident level variables			
Gun used			
Yes	4 (1.1)	41 (61.2)	43 (28.3)
No	352 (98.9)	26 (38.8)	109 (71.7)
		p < .01	p < .01

(Continued)

TABLE 7.2   Relationship Dynamics, Threatening Behavior, and Abuse Characteristics (*Continued*)

	Controls (n = 356) n (%)	Femicide W/ Suicide (n = 67) n (%)	Femicide W/O Suicide (n = 152) n (%)
Partner used alcohol or drugs			
Yes	123 (34.6)	42 (62.7)	90 (59.2)
No	233 (65.4)	25 (37.3)	62 (40.8)
		p < .01	**p < .01**
Victim used alcohol or drugs			
Yes	44 (12.4)	11 (16.4)	41 (27.0)
No	312 (87.6)	56 (83.6)	111 (73.0)
		p = .37	**p < .01**
Order of protection			
Yes	19 (5.3)	15 (22.4)	39 (25.7)
No	337 (94.7)	52 (77.6)	113 (74.3)
		p < .01	**p < .01**
Trigger—jealousy			
Yes	56 (15.7)	34 (50.7)	51 (33.6)
No	300 (84.3)	33 (49.3)	101 (66.4)
		p < .01	**p < .01**
Trigger—woman leaving			
Yes	34 (9.6)	21 (31.3)	51 (33.6)
No	322 (90.4)	46 (68.7)	101 (66.4)
		p < .01	**p < .01**
Trigger—woman has new relationship			
Yes	8 (2.2)	12 (17.9)	14 (9.2)
No	348 (97.8)	55 (82.1)	138 (90.8)
		p < .01	**p < .01**

Note: Unless otherwise noted, the referent time period for risk variables was the year prior to the most abusive event for controls and the year prior to the femicide for the femicide cases. *p* values are for comparisons between femicide group (with or without suicide) and controls based on chi-square tests for categorical variables and independent *t* tests for continuous variables; *p* values less than .05 are in boldface.

(56% versus 5%), threat(s) to take the children (20% versus 11%) and stalking behavior (24% versus 6%).

Characteristics of Physical Violence

Physical violence was reported to have increased in frequency and severity among femicide-suicide cases more often than among controls (59% versus 26% for frequency and 56% versus 20% for severity; Table 7.2). Choking/strangulation (52% versus 12%) and forced sex (57% versus 15%) were also more common among femicide-suicide cases.

Incident

Circumstances and triggers of the "worst battering episode" for controls and the killing event for femicide-suicide differed significantly (Table 7.2). Partner use of alcohol or drugs at the time of the incident was more common among femicide-suicide cases (63% versus 35%) as was the use of a gun (61% versus 1%). An order of protection was reported in 22% of the femicide-suicide cases versus in 5% of the controls. The triggers of jealousy (51% versus 16%), the woman leaving (31% versus 10%) and the woman having a new relationship (18% versus 2%) were all more common in the femicide-suicide incidents.

Regression Analyses

Regression analyses results are listed in Table 7.3. In the first logistic regression model examining sociodemographics (Model 1), a victim with less than high school (aOR = 4.0) or some college/trade school (aOR = 3.3), abuser with less than high school education (aOR = 3.8), abuser unemployed and not looking for a job (aOR = 2.7), and older abuser age (aOR = 1.1) were all independently associated with femicide-suicide risk. However, model 1 had little explanatory power with an R^2 = 0.16. Victim age and employment were not significant predictors of femicide-suicide, nor were race or ethnicity of the victim or abuser.

In the second logistic regression in which hypothesized risk factors for general violence were entered (Model 2), victim without a high school diploma (aOR = 3.1) and abuser unemployed not looking for a job (aOR = 2.9) from Model 1 remained significant predictors. Abuser gun access (aOR = 17.3) and abuser prior suicide threat(s) (aOR = 3.0) were added. Model 2 explanatory power increased to R^2 = 0.40. Victim mental health and prior suicide threat(s) and the abuser's problem alcohol drinking, illicit drug use, and prior arrest for a violence crime were not significant predictors.

The next group of variables examined characteristics of the intimate relationship (Model 3). In Model 3, six variables were significant, three from the prior model and three new variables: abuser unemployed not looking for a job (aOR = 3.3), abuser prior suicide threat(s) (aOR = 2.6), abuser gun access (aOR = 24.8), marital status of married (although not necessarily "together" at the time; aOR = 3.0); having a child of another man living in the home (aOR = 2.8), and having lived together in the past year but not prior to the worst incident (aOR = 2.8). The model R^2 increased to 0.51. The age difference between each woman and her abuser was not a significant predictor.

Relationship abuse dynamics were examined next (Model 4). Although a highly controlling abuser was a significant predictor (aOR = 5.0), the variance explained by the model was unchanged.

TABLE 7.3 Adjusted Odds Ratios (e^B) for IP Femicide-Suicide Risk Factors Among Women in a Physically Abusive Intimate Relationship

	Model 1	Model 2	Model 3	Model 4	Model 5/6	Model 7
Sociodemographic variables						
Abuser age (years)	1.1	ns				
Abuser education:						
< High school graduate	3.8	ns				
Abuser job status						
Unemployed, not seeking a job	2.7	2.9	3.3	ns		
Victim education						
< High school graduate	4.0	3.1	ns			
Some college	3.3	ns				
General violence variables						
Abuser threatened suicide		3.0	2.6	ns		
Abuser access to gun		17.3	24.8	14.5	13.0	ns
Relationship variables						
Married			3.0	3.6	2.9	ns
Cohabitation (reference: living together during entire past year)						
Previously lived together, separated prior to worst incident			2.8	3.9	4.3	ns
Victim had stepchild by another man			2.8	2.2	3.1	8.1
Abuse dynamics variables						
High control				5.0	ns	
Threatening behavior variables						
Threaten victim w/weapon					9.3	17.6
Threaten to kill victim					5.4	ns
Incident level variables						
Abuser used gun						161.1
Trigger—partner jealousy						3.8
Trigger—victim in a new relationship						15.8

Note: ns = not statistically significant; education reference group is college graduate; job status reference group is employed full time.

Threatening behaviors were examined next (Model 5). Six variables were significant in Model 5 including two threat variables: abuser gun access (aOR = 13.0), marriage (aOR = 2.9), having lived together in the past year but subsequently separated (aOR = 4.3), having a child of another man living in the home (aOR = 3.1), prior abuser threat(s) to kill the woman (aOR = 5.4) and prior abuser threat(s) with a weapon (aOR = 9.3). The model R^2 increased to 0.64. Despite highly significant bivariate relationships between physical violence variables and groups (femicide-suicide and controls), none remained significant when entered into the regression model (Model 6).

The final group of variables (Model 7) concerned the femicide-suicide event or the "worst battering episode" for the controls. In the final model, five variables were significant and explained 71% of the variance: child of another man living in the home (aOR = 8.1), prior abuser threats with a weapon (aOR = 17.6), the use of a gun in the event (aOR = 16.1), abusive incident triggers of the woman having a new relationship (aOR = 15.8), and abuser jealousy (aOR = 3.8).

DISCUSSION

The most important risk factor for intimate partner femicide-suicide is prior domestic violence against the victim. We found a higher proportion (72%) of prior domestic violence among femicide-suicide cases than has been reported by others (Bourget et al., 2000; Campanelli & Gilson, (2002); Morton et al., 1998), perhaps because we interviewed proxy informants rather than having to rely on criminal justice records only. The patterns of prior domestic violence were similar between the femicide-suicide and femicide without suicide relationships, with similar proportions of increase in severity and frequency, prior forced sex, strangulation/choking, and stalking. The only difference in prior domestic violence among our femicide-suicide cases was a smaller proportion of cases abused during pregnancy.

Significant explanatory power was achieved in identifying risk factors over and above domestic violence prior to the event for femicide-suicide and for event-level characteristics. Most notable among the risk factors that could be identifiable in encounters prior to the event (Model 5/6), based on magnitude of the odds ratio, were partner access to a gun, prior threats with a weapon, prior threats to kill her, estrangement from the perpetrator, a stepchild in the household, and a marital relationship. In the final incident level model (Model 7), even more explanatory power was achieved, with the use of a gun strongly predicting the femicide-suicide over the worst incident in an abusive relationship.

The use of a gun among the femicide-suicide cases (61%) is also strik-ing in that it is differentiated not only from the controls (1%) but from the femicide without suicide cases as well (28%). Bourget et al. (2000) reported similar findings in a sample of conjugal homicide-suicides in Quebec, where a gun was used in 61% of homicide-suicides versus 27% of homicides with-out suicides. Lund and Smorodinsky (2001) reporting from California and Easteal (1994) from Australia also found gun use significantly higher among homicide-suicides compared to homicides without suicide.

Two risk factors emerged in these models that were unique to femi-cide-suicide cases compared to overall femicide risk analyses and include: prior perpetrator suicide threats and victims having ever been married to the perpetrator. The importance of relationship variables and perpetrator characteristics in the study of the patterns of femicide-suicide is suggested by similar findings in older couples. In a study of older married male per-petrators of femicide followed by suicide, investigators found that the men, most of whom had a medical condition, failed to receive treatment for de-pression or received inappropriate antianxiety medications (Cohen, 2004). The availability, accessibility, and effectiveness of mental health services for men are an important issue for reducing the risk of femicide-suicide in the context of an abusive partner with depressive symptoms. An important risk factor in the overall femicide analyses that did not emerge as a significant independent predictor of femicide-suicide was perpetrator illicit drug use. However, still 50% of femicide-suicide perpetrators were reported to use illicit drugs.

It is also important to note that these cases of femicide-suicide differ in important ways from the more usual picture of intimate partner femicides of women as well as from less lethal intimate partner violence cases, as demon-strated in Tables 7.1 and 7.2. The femicide-suicide cases have higher propor-tions of White, Hispanic, and Asian victims and perpetrators, while African Americans had higher proportions in the femicide without suicide group. Even so, there were more African American perpetrators among the femi-cide-suicide cases with prior domestic violence than among the controls. The femicide-suicide cases were more likely to be married, employed, and report less illicit drug use and abuse during pregnancy. These differences suggest that practitioners working with domestic violence victims need to be aware that men who end up killing their wives (or girlfriends or estranged partners) and then themselves may have a larger "stake in conformity" than those who more usually kill their female intimate partners. In other words, they may appear to be a somewhat less dangerous domestic violence perpetrator than others who are seen in the domestic violence systems. Even so, the femicide-suicide perpetrators and femicide-only perpetrators had a similar background in terms of prior arrest for violent crimes (18% and 23% respectively) and they engendered a similar amount of fear in their partners (thinking their partner was capable of killing her, 53% and 49% respectively).

This study had some important limitations. In some cases proxy informants may not have been confidants. Even among confidants, behaviors may be over- or underreported (Koziol-McLain, Webster, & Campbell, 2001). Setting "don't know" to "no" responses for our regression analysis is likely to have muted our odds ratios. The sample size, though large considering femicide-suicide is relatively rare, was small for multivariate analysis—especially considering the large pool of variables—and did not allow for the examination of interactions. In some cases regression models were explored entering one variable at a time to avoid overfitting. We focused on p values in this report; confidence intervals and prediction rules would also be useful. For example, the 95% confidence interval for the prior perpetrator suicide threat estimated odds ratio (aOR = 2.6) in Model 3 (prior to entering abuse dynamics) was 1.2 to 5.9. That model (Model 3) correctly predicted 58% of the femicide-suicides in the sample. Future research is needed exploring the killing of other family members such as children, which occurred in 40 of our 310 study cases.

These study findings have important implications. First, for policy makers, access and use of guns significantly increases the risk of death for both victims and abusive partners. It is therefore particularly important that those perpetrators with a prior domestic violence or other violent crime conviction are prevented from gun ownership and any guns they own are removed at the time of adjudication of the crime as is mandated by federal law. Second, many of the significant risk factors for femicide-suicide involve characteristics of the abusive partner. Health professionals, especially in mental health and alcohol and drug treatment programs, should assess for dangerousness, asking men about past abusive behaviors toward their intimate partner, suicidal ideation, and depression—especially in the context of separating from their partner. Verbalization of extreme jealousy, accusations that their partner is having a sexual relationship with a different partner, making statements like, "If I can't have her nobody can" or "Can't live with her; can't live without her" should all be taken extremely seriously if there is any evidence of prior violence. Third, women who disclose violence in their relationship and are considering separating from their partner should receive individualized interventions including assessment of dangerousness with a knowledgeable practitioner, referral to domestic violence advocacy services, offer to call the criminal justice authorities, and safety planning. The femicide-suicide risk factors identified in this analysis (with the exception of marital status) are included in the revised Danger Assessment instrument (Campbell, 2005a, 2005b). While there is significant overlap in femicide and femicide followed by suicide risk factors—especially for the strongest predictors—important differences were detected, thus signaling a need for continued theoretical development and empirical investigation.

Acknowledgments. The authors thank the other participating members of the femicide research team including Doris Campbell, Mary Ann Curry, Faye Gary, Carolyn Sachs, Phyllis Sharps, Susan Wilt, Victoria Fry, Jennifer Manganello, Xiao Xu, Jo Ellen Stinchcomb, and Janet Schollenberger. We also thank our advocacy, criminal justice, and medical examiner collaborators in each of the study sites, such as Richard C. Harruff, MD, PhD, Chief Medical Examiner King County; and Arthur Kellerman, MD, for his consultation. This research was supported by joint funding from the National Institute on Alcohol Abuse and Alcoholism, National Institute on Drug Abuse, National Institute of Mental Health, National Institutes on Aging, Centers for Disease Control and Prevention, and National Institute of Justice, principal investigator Jacquelyn Campbell, PhD, RN (RO1 DA/AA 11156). The National Institute of Mental Health also supported Jane Koziol-McLain, PhD, RN, in a postdoctoral fellowship at Johns Hopkins University (T32 MH20014).

REFERENCES

Aderibigbe, Y. A. (1997). Violence in America: A survey of suicide linked to homicides. *Journal of Forensic Science, 42*(4), 662–665.

Allen, N. H. (1983). Homicide followed by suicide: Los Angeles, 1970–1979. *Suicide and Life-Threatening Behavior, 13*(3), 155–165.

Barraclough, B., & Harris, E. C. (2002). Suicide preceded by murder: The epidemiology of homicide-suicide in England and Wales 1988–92. *Psychological Medicine, 32*(4), 577–584.

Belfrage, H., & Rying, M. (2004). Characteristics of spousal homicide perpetrators: A study of all cases of spousal homicide in Sweden 1990–1999. *Criminal Behavior & Mental Health, 14*(2), 121–133.

Bourget, D., Gagne, P., & Moamai, J. (2000). Spousal homicide and suicide in Quebec. *Journal of American Academic Psychiatry Law, 28*(2), 179–182.

Brock, K. (2002). *American roulette: The untold story of murder-suicide in the United States.* Washington, DC: Violence Policy Center.

Buteau, J., Lesage, A. D., & Kiely, M. C. (1993). Homicide followed by suicide: A Quebec case series, 1988–1990. *Canadian Journal of Psychiatry, 38*(8), 552–556.

Campanelli, C., & Gilson, T. (2002). Murder-suicide in New Hampshire, 1995–2000. *American Journal of Forensic Medical Pathology, 23*(3), 248–251.

Campbell, J. C. (1995). Prediction of homicide of and by battered women. In J. C. Campbell (Ed.), *Assessing the risk of dangerousness: Potential for further violence of sexual offenders, batterers, and child abusers* (pp. 93–113). Newbury Park, CA: Sage.

Campbell, J. C. (2005a). *Psychometric data: Danger assessment.* Retrieved October 2005, from http://www.dangerassessment.org

Campbell, J. C. (2005b). Commentary on Websdale: Lethality assessment approaches: Reflections on their use and ways forward. *Violence Against Women, 11*(9), 1206–1213.

Campbell, J. C., Webster, D., Koziol-McLain, J., Block, C., Campbell, D., Curry, M. A., et al. (2003). Risk factors for femicide in abusive relationships: Results from a multisite case control study. *American Journal of Public Health, 93*(7), 1089–1097.

Chan, C. Y., Beh, S. L., & Broadburst, R. G. (2004). Homicide-suicide in Hong Kong, 1989–1998. *Forensic Science International, 140*(2–3), 261–267.

Cohen, D. (2004). Homicide-suicide in older people. *Psychiatric Times, 17*(1).

Cohen, D., Llorente, M., & Eisdorfer, C. (1998). Homicide-suicide in older persons. *American Journal of Psychiatry, 155*(3), 390–396.

Cooper, M., & Eaves, D. (1996). Suicide following homicide in the family. *Violence and Victims, 11*(2), 99–112.

Currens, S., Tritsch, T., Jones, D., Bush, G., Vance, J., Frederick, K., et al. (1991). Current trends homicide followed by suicide—Kentucky, 1985–1990. *Morbidity Mortality Weekly Report, 40*(38), 652–653, 659.

Dawson, M. (2005). Intimate femicide followed by suicide: Examining the role of premeditation. *Suicide and Life-Threatening Behavior, 35*(1), 76–90.

Dawson, R., & Gartner, R. (1998a). Differences in the characteristics of intimate femicides: The role of relationship state and relationship status. *Homicide Studies, 2*, 378–399.

Dawson, M., & Gartner, R. (1998b). *Male proprietariness or despair? Examining the gendered nature of homicides followed by suicides.* Paper presented at the American Society of Criminology, Washington, DC.

Easteal, P. (1994). Homicide-suicides between adult sexual intimates: An Australian study. *Suicide and Life-Threatening Behavior, 24*(2), 140–151.

Easteal, P. W. (1993). *Killing the beloved.* Canberra: Australian Institute of Criminology.

Felthous, A. R., & Hempel, A. (1995). Combined homicide-suicides: A review. *Journal of Forensic Sciences, 40*(5), 846–857.

Gillespie, M., Hearn, V., & Silverman, R. A. (1998). Suicide following homicide in Canada. *Homicide Studies, 2*(1), 46–63.

Hannah, S. G., Turf, E. E., & Fierro, M. F. (1998). Murder-suicide in central Virginia: A descriptive epidemiologic study and empiric validation of the Hanzlick-Koponen typology. *American Journal of Forensic Medical Pathology, 19*(3), 275–283.

Hillbrand, M. (2002). *Integrated assessment of suicide and homicide risk.* Retrieved June 9, 2003, from http://www.apa.org/divisions/div12/sections/section7/news/sp02/hillbrand_sp02.html

Johnson, H., & Hotton, T. (2003). Losing control: Homicide risk in estranged and intact intimate relationships. *Homicide Studies, 7*(1), 58–84.

Koziol-McLain, J., Webster, D., & Campbell, J. C. (2001). Attempted homicide victim and proxy reports of intimate-partner homicide risk factors: Do they agree? In P. H. Blackman & V. L. Leggett (Eds.), *The diversity of homicide: Proceedings of the 2000 Annual Meeting of the Homicide Research Working Group* (pp. 111–116). Washington, DC: Federal Bureau of Investigation.

Lecomte, D., & Fornes, P. (1998). Homicide followed by suicide: Paris and its suburbs, 1991–1996. *Journal of Forensic Science, 43*(4), 760–764.

Lund, L. E., & Smorodinsky, S. (2001). Violent death among intimate partners: A comparison of homicide and homicide followed by suicide in California. *Suicide and Life-Threatening Behavior, 31*(4), 451–459.

Malphurs, J. E., & Cohen, D. (2002). A newspaper surveillance study of homicide-suicide in the United States. *American Journal of Forensic Medical Pathology, 23*(2), 142–148.

Malphurs, J. E., & Cohen, D. (2005). A statewide case-control study of spousal homicide-suicide in older persons. *American Journal of Geriatric Psychiatry, 13*(3), 211–217.

Malphurs, J. E., Eisdorfer, C., & Cohen, D. (2001). A comparison of antecedents of homicide-suicide and suicide in older married men. *American Journal of Geriatric Psychiatry, 9*(1), 49–57.

Marzuk, P. M., Tardiff, K., & Hirsch, C. S. (1992). The epidemiology of murder-suicide. *Journal of the American Medical Association, 267*(23), 3179–3183.

Milroy, C. M., Dratsas, M., & Ranson, D. L. (1997). Homicide-suicide in Victoria, Australia. *American Journal of Forensic Medical Pathology, 18*(4), 369–373.

Morton, E., Runyan, C. W., Moracco, K. E., & Butts, J. (1998). Partner homicide-suicide involving female homicide victims: A population-based study in North Carolina, 1988–1992. *Violence and Victims, 13*(2), 91–106.

National Center for Injury Prevention and Control CDC. (2005). Homicide and suicide rates—national violent death reporting system, six states, 2003. *Morbidity Mortality Weekly Report, 54*(15), 377–380.

Palermo, G. B., Smith, M. B., Jentzen, J. M., Henry, T. E., Konicek, P. J., Peterson, G. F., et al. (1997). Murder-suicide of the jealous paranoia type: A multicenter statistical pilot study. *American Journal of Forensic Medical Pathology, 18*(4), 374–383.

Paulozzi, L. J., Mercy, J., Frazier, L., Jr., & Annest, J. L. (2004). CDC's National Violent Death Reporting System: Background and methodology. *Injury Prevention, 10*(1), 47–52.

Polk, K. (1994). *When men kill: Scenarios of masculine violence.* Cambridge, UK: Cambridge University Press.

Rosenbaum, M. (1990). The role of depression in couples involved in murder-suicide and homicide. *American Journal of Psychiatry, 147*(8), 1036–1039.

SPSS. (2001). *Advanced techniques: Regression.* Chicago, IL: SPSS Inc.

Stack, S. (1997). Homicide followed by suicide: An analysis of Chicago data. *Criminology, 35*(3), 435–453.

Walsh, S., & Hemenway, D. (2005). Intimate partner violence: Homicides followed by suicides in Kentucky. *Journal of the Kentucky Medical Association, 103*(1), 10–13.

Websdale, N. (1999). *Understanding domestic homicide*. Boston: Northeastern University Press.

Wilson, M., & Daly, M. (1993a). An evolutionary psychological perspective on male sexual proprietariness and violence against wives. *Violence and Victims, 8*, 271–294.

Wilson, M., & Daly, M. (1993b). Spousal homicide risk and estrangement. *Violence and Victims, 8*(1), 3–15.

Wolfgang, M. E. (1958). An analysis of homicide-suicide. *Journal of Clinical and Experimental Psychopathology, 19*(3), 208–218.

Author Index

Index

DANGERASSESSMENT.ORG

An online training program for intimate partner risk assessment

Q: **How do you identify the domestic violence victims in the most danger?**

A: **Become a DANGER ASSESSMENT Certified Assessor**

The Danger Assessment, an evaluation tool developed by **Jacquelyn Campbell, PhD, RN, FAAN**, is for those involved with domestic violence cases. It has been used and validated by:

Law Enforcement Professionals • Healthcare Professionals
Domestic Violence Advocates • Social Workers

*Train at your own pace

*Earn a personalized Danger Assessor certificate

*Receive the guide for interpreting the Danger Assessment tool

Go to
WWW.DANGERASSESSMENT.ORG

Info@DANGERASSESSMENT.ORG

Every year, 3-4 million women in the US are abused and 1200-1500 are killed by their abusers.

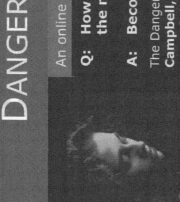

THE INSTITUTE FOR **JOHNS HOPKINS NURSING**
JOHNS HOPKINS UNIVERSITY
SCHOOL OF **NURSING**